T0188871

Register Now for Online Access to Your Book!

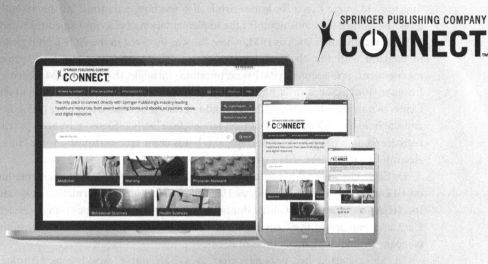

SPRINGER PUBLISHING COMPANY

CONNECT™

Your print purchase of *Project Management for the Advanced Practice Nurse, Second Edition* **includes online access to the contents of your book**—increasing accessibility, portability, and searchability!

Access today at:

http://connect.springerpub.com/content/book/978-0-8261-6196-3 or scan the QR code at the right with your smartphone and enter the access code below.

P2ELK3T8

Scan here for quick access.

If you are experiencing problems accessing the digital component of this product, please contact our customer service department at cs@springerpub.com

The online access with your print purchase is available at the publisher's discretion and may be removed at any time without notice.

Publisher's Note: New and used products purchased from third-party sellers are not guaranteed for quality, authenticity, or access to any included digital components.

SPC

SPRINGER / PUBLISHING COMPANY

View all our products at springerpub.com

Carolyn Sipes, PhD, CNS, APRN, PMP, RN-BC, NEA-BC, FAAN, is a professor for DNP and PhD programs; she was formerly a professor for the Nursing Informatics Specialty Track. Dr. Sipes has more than 35 years' experience in management, as a director and nurse executive leader, while also teaching part time. At the executive level, she worked as a consultant for the implementation of electronic medical records (EMRs) at companies such as IBM, where she was involved in the iSOFT pilot project in England with the National Health Service (NHS), and completed her project management professional (PMP) certification through the Project Management Institute (PMI). She also is board certified by the American Nurses Credentialing Center in nursing informatics (RN-BC) and as an advanced nurse executive (NEA-BC), and she holds a PhD as well as clinical nurse specialist (CNS) and advanced practice registered nurse (APRN) licenses. She also holds eight Epic certifications for clinical electronic health record (EHR) implementation.

Dr. Sipes has worked as a senior/principal consultant on 23 EMR implementations over 12 years for such companies as HealthLink, Healthcare Informatics Associates, Inc. (HIA), and Cleveland Clinic Abu Dhabi, to name a few. Dr. Sipes is the president, CEO, and founder of the Center for EHR Program Management, LLC, a consulting company for the implementations of EHRs.

Dr. Sipes started her nursing career as a BSN nurse, working in neurology/neurosurgery, then completed her MSN and CNS in Chicago, and then worked as a pediatric CNS and as an NIH study coordinator for pediatric AIDS. She received an NIH fellowship to complete her doctoral studies in HIV/AIDS at Rush University, Chicago. During this time, she also worked as a director of outcomes research and designed the Medical Outcomes System Assessment (MOS) tool to evaluate physical functional assessments for subacute care organizations. Her dissertation on male caregivers who provided care for their partners with HIV/AIDS has been published and updated numerous times. During this time, she also served as the vice president of an HIV/AIDS clinic in Chicago. After completing her doctorate, she worked as a research scientist for a major pharmaceutical company, where she designed the Tolerability of Medication Assessment (TOMA) tool. The research conducted using this tool was presented at the World AIDS Conference in Barcelona, Spain. She has authored numerous publications on project management as well as informatics competencies and has presented research papers nationally and internationally, including at the 2016 Nursing Informatics World Nursing Conference in Geneva, Switzerland.

Dr. Sipes began designing and teaching informatics courses while consulting as a full-time senior project manager/director. These experiences led her to teaching informatics full time at the master's and doctoral levels. She has also published and presented, nationally and internationally, more than 35 nursing informatics and project management topics, including webinars at the American Association of Critical-Care Nurses (AACN), and is on the national American Nurses Association (ANA) 2019 Workgroup to revise the nursing informatics scope and standards of practice. She is a fellow of the American Academy of Nursing.

PROJECT MANAGEMENT FOR THE ADVANCED PRACTICE NURSE

Second Edition

Carolyn Sipes, PhD, CNS, APRN, PMP, RN-BC, NEA-BC, FAAN

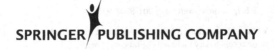

SPRINGER PUBLISHING COMPANY

Springer Publishing Company, LLC
11 West 42nd Street
New York, NY 10036
www.springerpub.com
http://connect.springerpub.com

Acquisitions Editor: Joseph Morita
Compositor: Amnet Systems

ISBN: 978-0-8261-6195-6
ebook ISBN: 978-0-8261-6196-3
Instructor's Manual ISBN: 978-0-8261-6429-2
Instructor's PowerPoints ISBN: 978-0-8261-6428-5
DOI: 10.1891/9780826161963

Instructor's Materials: Qualified instructors may request supplements by emailing textbook@springerpub .com

19 20 21 22/5 4 3 2 1

The author and the publisher of this Work have made every effort to use sources believed to be reliable to provide information that is accurate and compatible with the standards generally accepted at the time of publication. Because medical science is continually advancing, our knowledge base continues to expand. Therefore, as new information becomes available, changes in procedures become necessary. We recommend that the reader always consult current research and specific institutional policies before performing any clinical procedure. The author and publisher shall not be liable for any special, consequential, or exemplary damages resulting, in whole or in part, from the readers' use of, or reliance on, the information contained in this book. The publisher has no responsibility for the persistence or accuracy of URLs for external or third-party Internet websites referred to in this publication and does not guarantee that any content on such websites is, or will remain, accurate or appropriate.

Library of Congress Cataloging-in-Publication Data

Names: Sipes, Carolyn, author.
Title: Project management for the advanced practice nurse / Carolyn Sipes.
Description: Second edition. | New York, NY : Springer Publishing Company,
   [2020] | Includes bibliographical references and index.
Identifiers: LCCN 2019010266 (print) | LCCN 2019011510 (ebook) | ISBN
   9780826161963 (eBook) | ISBN 9780826161956 (print : alk. paper) | ISBN
   9780826161963 (e-book) | ISBN 9780826164292 (instructor's manual) | ISBN
   9780826164285 (instructor's Powerpoints)
Subjects: | MESH: Advanced Practice Nursing—organization & administration |
   Program Development | Planning Techniques
Classification: LCC RT41 (ebook) | LCC RT41 (print) | NLM WY 128 | DDC
   610.73—dc23
LC record available at https://lccn.loc.gov/2019010266

Carolyn Sipes: https://orcid.org/0000-0001-8708-9359

Printed in the United States of America.

CONTENTS

CONTRIBUTORS

Toni Hebda, PhD, MNEd, MSIS, RN-C, Professor, MSN Program, Chamberlain College of Nursing, Downers Grove, Illinois

Tracy Stogner, DNP, APRN, RN, PMHCNS-BC, Curriculum Technology Manager MSN-ST and Visiting Professor RN-BSN, Chamberlain College of Nursing, Downers Grove, Illinois

Susan Waltz, DNP, MSN, RN, CNE, Associate Professor, MSN Program, Chamberlain College of Nursing, Downers Grove, Illinois

FOREWORD

Project management is an important skill in both career and life, yet little has been written to provide nurses and other healthcare professionals acting in leadership and advanced practice roles with the tools needed to ensure success in this area. The lack of literature and texts serves neither educators nor healthcare professionals well and has forced them to draw from other disciplines—until now, with the culmination of this book.

In part, the lack of project management literature may be attributed to its fairly recent definition as well as confusion over its defining characteristics and how those characteristics distinguish it from other aspects of management. According to the Project Management Institute (PMI), project management is "the application of knowledge, skills, tools, and techniques to project activities to meet the project requirements" (2017, p. 10). Project management consists of five phases—initiation, planning, implementing/executing, monitoring and controlling, and closing. Projects differ from other activities because of their temporary nature and intent to create a unique product or service.

PMI also sought to establish project management as a profession, although it is not necessary to formally assume that role to benefit and apply associated knowledge and skills, as will be demonstrated through the many examples provided in this book. It is my contention that project management skills will play a key role in the collaborative transformation of the healthcare delivery system through the efforts of engaged healthcare professionals, payors, and consumers via a multitude of projects over time. *The Future of Nursing* report (Institute of Medicine [IOM], 2010) specifically calls for nurses to play a pivotal role in transformation. One tool to achieve transformation is information technology. The implementation of any information technology in a given healthcare organization exemplifies a project. Nursing informatics as a specialty delineates project management as key to its work. The American Nurses Credentialing Center's (2018) test content outline for the informatics nursing credentialing examination includes all facets of project management. As a long-time nurse educator and coauthor of *Handbook of Informatics for Nurses and Health Care Professionals*, I recognize the importance of project management to successful outcomes and particularly to the integration of information systems and technology.

This book offers guidance and insights and ties the skills of a seasoned project manager, advanced practice nurse, and nurse educator together to take the reader through all phases of the project management process from start to finish through tools integrated throughout the text.

Toni Hebda, PhD, MNEd, MSIS, RN-C
Professor, MSN Program
Chamberlain College of Nursing
Downers Grove, Illinois

REFERENCES

American Nurses Credentialing Center. (2018). *Test content outline*. Retrieved from https://www.nursingworld.org/~490a5b/globalassets/certification/certification-specialty-pages/resources/test-content-outlines/27-tco-rds-2016-effective-date-march-23-2018_100317.pdf

Institute of Medicine. (2010). *The future of nursing: Leading change, advancing health*. Washington, DC: National Academies Press. Retrieved from http://books.nap.edu

Project Management Institute, Inc. (2017). *A guide to the project management body of knowledge (PMBOK guide)* (6th ed., p. 10). Newtown Square, PA: Author.

PREFACE

The second edition of this book continues to grow from teaching and practice experiences in nursing informatics as well as from working as a consultant and project manager (PM) implementing electronic health records (EHRs) nationally and internationally. Concepts in this text provide a guiding framework that graduate students can use in both clinical practice and leadership, as well as when preparing a practicum assignment for graduation and residencies to guide MSN, nurse executive (NE), and doctoral projects such as those in DNP and PhD programs. This author continues to observe what nurses consider as only project management and business-related skills not related to nursing practice, but which in fact are basic organizational skills needed by *all nurses*. Professionals are expected to have these skills and use them during the project management process, which is basically similar to the nursing process in design/ creating, planning, implementing, monitoring and controlling, and evaluation competencies. Nurses are greatly skilled at managing patient care and outcomes but fail to connect the dots of project management and the nursing processes, stating it does not apply to them.

This book endeavors to support nurses and healthcare professionals in understanding and applying project management (nursing process) structures to goals and objectives that must be accomplished in an organized way, thus promoting the development of leadership skills as well. It outlines the phases of project management, such as design and planning, implementation, monitoring and controlling, and final evaluation. Tools utilized in the process include timelines and tracking tools, and many other management documents that help application and monitoring tasks are included.

This book is organized into three sections, following the convention of project management standards originally developed in the 1950s by engineers in an effort to manage the chaos of projects. Although based on proven concepts and standards, this book is focused on defining concepts in a way that non-PMs, such as advanced practice registered nurses (APRNs), DNPs, clinical practitioners, research nurses (PhDs), and other interprofessional clinicians and teams, can more easily follow in order to apply organizational processes, considered business operations of a healthcare organization, to clinical practice. More frequently in today's practice, APRNs, DNPs, and PhDs and other interprofessional teams are expected to apply these same concepts when managing their own practices. These concepts are also included in the American Nurses Association's (ANA) *Nursing Informatics Scope and Standards of Practice* (2015, pp. 68–92) as expectations of practice.

New to the second edition are case scenarios with exemplars of a process or application of a tool, critical thinking questions and activities, and new, updated content based on the current practices and national organizations' mandates. Many tools used in organizations for management of goals and objectives are included in each chapter. *Qualified instructors may obtain access to supplementary material (Instructor's Manual and PowerPoints) by emailing textbook@springerpub.com.*

Each chapter provides information related to the five basic concepts of project management, including details outlining the skills and knowledge expectations, tools, and techniques needed to accomplish goals and objectives using an organizing framework.

- *Section I:* Chapter 1, Basic Project Management for Advanced Practice Nurses and Healthcare Professionals, includes the key concepts and definitions of the key competency areas an APRN as PM should know. Constraints are defined, as are project steps and APRN role descriptions.

- Chapter 2, Advanced Practice Nurse Role Descriptions and Application of Project Management Concepts, lists some of the common roles an APRN might assume and includes sample job descriptions for which project management skills are required.

- *Section II*: Chapter 3, Design/Initiation: Project Management— Phase 1, includes descriptions of what to do first, such as a project's design and planning steps, gap and workflow analysis, team and system selection, work breakdown structure, creating a responsibility matrix, understanding team behaviors, and developing a project charter and scope, as well as other necessary management documents and tools.

- Chapter 4, Planning: Project Management—Phase 2, explains the steps to take when developing a project plan, network diagram, risk management plan, communication plan, change management plan, kick-off meeting, and project launch.

■ Chapter 5, Implementation/Execution—Phase 3, explains supervision and implementation, which comprise the longest phase in a project and include processes for implementing the plans developed in the previous steps. Status reports and tracking tools become a critical component of implementation, as do other elements of quality control, such as testing and go-live processes.

■ Chapter 6, Monitoring and Controlling: Project Management—Phase 4, describes the monitoring and control steps and defines the processes and tools needed to track the implementation, performance assessment, and dashboard reports, while controlling budgets and resources.

■ Chapter 7, Closing the Project—Phase 5, outlines the concluding and closing steps of the project management process and explains how to do the verification audit using the audit tool; how to conduct a lessons-learned assessment that verifies all processes are complete; how to arrange for postimplementation assessment and follow-up; and, finally, formal sign-off by all steering committees, sponsors, stakeholders, and leadership.

■ *Section III*: Chapter 8, Case Studies: Applying Project Management Concepts and Tools, includes exemplars of how and where the APRN, DNP, chief nurse informatics officer (CNIO), clinical nurse specialist (CNS), nurse practitioner (NP), and others might apply the concepts of project management to their everyday practice.

While this text is not inclusive of every detail required for a project, it is based on over 20 years of experience managing different types of projects. However, there are basic concepts that have never changed, including the standards of practice and the guiding framework for project management—design/planning, implementation, monitoring and control, and final evaluation.

Carolyn Sipes

REFERENCE

American Nurses Association. (2015). *Nursing informatics scope and standards of practice*. Silver Spring, MD: Nursesbooks.org.

ACKNOWLEDGMENTS

I am deeply grateful for the love, patience, continued encouragement, and support of my husband, Jim, and my family, Chris, Doug, and Susan, and their families.

I am also extremely grateful for the ongoing support and continued encouragement of peer faculty at Chamberlain College of Nursing, MSN program—Professors Dr. Kathleen Hunter, Dr. Dee McGonigle, and Dr. Toni Hebda—and to all of the students who are always challenging and ask thought-provoking questions.

SECTION I

INTRODUCTION AND
ROLES OF THE ADVANCED
PRACTICE NURSE

CHAPTER 1

BASIC PROJECT MANAGEMENT FOR ADVANCED PRACTICE NURSES AND HEALTHCARE PROFESSIONALS

LEARNING OBJECTIVES

Upon completion of this chapter, the reader will be able to:

1. Discuss three driving forces that develop project management skills.
2. Discuss the history of project management.
3. Discuss why project management is needed.
4. List three principles of project management.
5. List two tasks that program management addresses.
6. Identify the constraints of project management outline.

OUTLINE

- Key Terms
- Introduction
- Examples of APRN Projects/Roles

- The Nursing Process and Project Management
- Definition of a Project
- What Is Project Management?
- Project Management Processes
- Principles of Project Management
- Project Management: Why Do We Need It?
- Summary

KEY TERMS

- American Association of Colleges of Nursing (AACN)
- American Nurses Association (ANA)
- Advanced practice registered nurse (APRN)
- Certified nurse-midwife (CNM)
- Certified nursing specialist (CNS)
- Certified registered nurse anesthetist (CRNA)
- Chief nursing officer (CNO)
- Doctor of nursing practice (DNP)
- Electronic health record (EHR)
- Informatics nurse specialist (INS)
- Nurse administrator (NA)
- Nurse informaticist (NI)
- Nurse practitioner (NP)
- Project manager (PM)
- Project management (PM)

INTRODUCTION

This chapter provides the introduction to the concepts of project management. You already know many of these, as they are basic to many other functions, such as the nursing process, which will be discussed later. The project management concepts you think of as only applicable to businesses and do not have anything to do with your practice are indeed relevant, as you will see as you move through this text. Other information in this chapter includes examples of the nursing roles that use the project management concepts, such as definitions and principles of the project management process, explanation why we need it, and exemplars of how and where it can be applied.

CASE SCENARIO 1.1

Amy has been working on the medical floor of St. Joe's Hospital for five years and is in the MSN program at the local university. She has completed her core courses and is now taking the final management courses. The chief nursing officer (CNO) has learned of Amy's career goals and wants her to be considered for promotion to nurse manager of the medical–surgical department. The CNO reminds Amy that in addition to completing the management courses, she will also have to choose and develop a practicum project before she graduates. The prospect of the project makes Amy very nervous; she indicates that she does not know how to do a project and has never done one.

The CNO encourages Amy and reminds her how she helped organize her sister's wedding last summer: how she helped to set a date, plan who would be there, select the invitations, arrange for the church, and all of the other details that go into planning a wedding. The CNO shares that her practicum will be a project with similar tasks, such as designing what she will do based on a health issue she would like to resolve. After this, Amy will then plan the necessary steps to complete the project, including setting end dates for completion, then after she has planned her project, she will need to implement it step by step and finally assess her results and determine what will need to be fixed or changed.

The CNO assures Amy that project management concepts in the practicum are the same processes found in the nursing practice. The five steps are the same for both processes—except that some of the terminologies are different—and the end point is the same. She also reminds Amy that her project has a starting point and an end point and that it will be short term, unlike some of the other projects the hospital has proposed, which take years to complete.

The CNO further assures Amy that she will be her mentor and that she also has developed and implemented many projects in the past as part of her CNO training and current leadership role responsibility. She will help Amy learn project management skills.

Before we get into the basics of project management, it is important to first understand how the process will affect advanced practice registered nurses (APRNs), including nurse practitioners (NPs), nurse executives (NEs), and many others like Amy, as well as other healthcare professionals, such as CNOs and chief nursing informatics officers (CNIOs). Chapter 1, Basic Project Management for Advanced Practice Nurses and Healthcare Professionals, and Chapter 2, Advanced Practice Nurse Role Descriptions and Application of Project Management Concepts, define some of the key roles assumed as project manager (PM) or when using project management skills in practice. The concepts are based on proven project management standards and terminology developed over decades of practice. This chapter focuses on defining concepts in a way that non-PMs, such as APRNs and other healthcare clinicians, will better understand definitions and processes in order to apply the concepts to practice.

According to the American Nurses Association (ANA), APRNs employ principles of project management where they are uniquely suited, because they have experience in information technology (IT) implementation, as they follow similar phases of the nursing process of assessment, diagnosis, planning, implementation, and evaluation (ANA, 2008, 2010, 2015). In the same sense, APRNs can be viewed as the "managers" of patient care, when applying similar processes to determine and achieve a specific outcome for patients.

This chapter is organized to define the similarities between the nursing process and project management. Basic project management definitions, processes, concepts, and plans are discussed and presented in Section II, Phases of Project Management. Similar to the nursing process, concepts of project management require that as a project or care plan is designed, planned, applied, and carried out, it is being supervised, regulated (or controlled), and then, finally, evaluated and ended/concluded. Chapter 2, Advanced Practice Nurse Role Descriptions and Application of Project Management Concepts, includes the different PM roles that might be applied by APRNs.

Section II, Phases of Project Management, describes each of the five phases of project management, defined with a list of the activities that occur in each phase. It also includes examples of the tools that are used in each step as well as a description of the content used in the documents that PMs develop.

Chapter 8, Case Studies: Applying Project Management Concepts and Tools, in Section III, Application of Project Management Concepts and Tools, provides case studies and exemplars that suggest how the APRN, NP, leadership and NE, doctor of nursing practice (DNP), and other healthcare professionals will use the various concepts of project management in different projects they might direct or when organizing a project they might need to develop in graduate school. Examples of project management are included for the roles of APRN as an administrator, certified nursing specialist (CNS), NP, chief nurse informatics officer (CNIO), or other levels of management in an organization.

> ▶ **QUESTIONS TO CONSIDER BEFORE READING ON**
>
> 1. What are some of the APRN roles most commonly found in practice today?
> 2. What are the other APRN roles to consider for the future?

EXAMPLES OF APRN PROJECTS/ROLES

According to a report by the American Association of Colleges of Nursing (AACN), an APRN can assume many different roles. A partial list includes working as:

- *NPs* who deliver frontline primary and acute care in community clinics, schools, hospitals, and other settings. They perform such services as diagnosing and treating common acute illnesses and injuries, providing immunizations, conducting physical exams, and managing high blood pressure, diabetes, and other chronic problems.

- *Certified nurse-midwives (CNMs)* who provide prenatal and gynecological care to normal healthy women; deliver babies in hospitals, private homes, and birthing centers; and continue with follow-up postpartum care.

- *CNSs* who provide care in a range of specialty areas, such as cardiac, oncology, neonatal, pediatric, and obstetric/gynecologic nursing, to name a few.

- *Certified registered nurse anesthetists (CRNAs)* who administer more than 65% of all anesthetics given to patients each year and are the sole providers of anesthesia in approximately one third of the U.S. hospitals (AACN, 2014).

These roles come to mind first when considering an APRN role, although there are many others, and roles continue to be revised, updated, and expanded. Any potential projects for an APRN would require knowledge and use of various project management skills presented in the following sections. Typically, an APRN would need the knowledge and skills in the following list to complete a graduate practicum, including the need to design, plan, implement, and then evaluate the final outcomes before graduation. Examples of project management knowledge and skills are discussed in later chapters. Examples of some of the project activities that APRNs have been involved in include:

- Evaluate a learning management system that has been implemented.
- Assess gaps in patients' needs and develop recommendations for practice.
- Assess the quality of how a particular process or program is functioning, and provide recommendations for improvement.
- Mentor other graduate students' development, and then recommend strategies for implementation of processes and programs to meet identified needs.
- Design and implement qualitative tools for data collection.
- Develop evidence-based practice guidelines for identified programs, such as wound management.
- Develop and conduct a needs assessment for a population of patients.
- Design and implement protocols for a hospital-wide program to address the identification, prevention, and treatment of skin tears.
- Design a potential suicide-tracking website and tracking devices for the military.

Examples of APRN roles are listed in Box 1.1. This is a partial list and will change as APRN roles are expanded and updated.

In addition to the roles listed in Box 1.1, DNPs maintain clinical practice, conduct program evaluations, implement practice changes and improvements, manage quality improvement, and translate evidence into practice. The difference between a PhD and DNP is that a PhD generates new knowledge and scientific discovery, although they still manage patients and clinics, whereas DNP is more clinical practice focused. Many DNP projects are listed on the website titled DNP Scholarly Projects: Archived and Searchable, which can be found at www.doctorsofnursing practice.org.

BOX 1.1

EXAMPLES OF ADVANCED PRACTICE NURSE ROLES
Clinical nurse specialist (CNS)
Certified registered nurse anesthetist (CRNA)
Certified nurse-midwife (CNM)
Chief nursing officer (CNO)
Chief nursing informatics officer (CNIO)
Doctor of nursing practice (DNP)
Director of advanced practice nursing
Informatics nurse specialist (INS)
Nurse administrator (NA)
Nurse informaticist (NI)
Nurse practitioner (NP)

SOURCE: Sipes, C. (2019). *Project management for the advanced practice nurse* (2nd ed.). New York, NY: Springer Publishing Company.

▶ **QUESTIONS TO CONSIDER BEFORE READING ON**
1. How are the project management and nursing processes similar?
2. Discuss four processes that are the same in both practices.
3. What is a project?
4. What is a constraint?

THE NURSING PROCESS AND PROJECT MANAGEMENT

Although the concept of project management seems foreign to many, there is a common thread that applies it to the different types of work that nurses do. That thread is the nursing process, one of the first core principles of nursing practice that nurses learn to use when delivering the best evidence-based patient care. The idea that nurses will understand and be able to apply the five basic principles of project management comes from its similarity to the five steps of the nursing process that are discussed in the previous sections. The steps are similar to some project management terms and tasks;

one just needs to learn the differences in semantics between the nursing process and project management concepts. However, nurses, especially as they achieve more advanced levels of practice, will find many similarities between the processes of project management and the nursing process— the main difference being that they are working with a project instead of patients. There are overlaps of the five processes throughout all of nursing. The five project management concepts are also listed as expectations for practice in the ANA *Scope and Standards of Practice for Nursing Informatics* (2015) as well as NEs (American Organization of Nurse Executives, 2015).

DEFINITION OF A PROJECT

A "project" is a planned set of interrelated tasks that need to be completed within a specific timeline. The specific beginning and ending dates define the temporary process that may last weeks and/or months but is not considered long term, such as the previous example of Amy planning her sister's wedding.

For example, many projects found in healthcare organizations today are related to installing a new electronic health record (EHR) system. These projects have a specific or dedicated PM who, working with a team, designs, plans, implements/builds, and evaluates an EHR, based on the skills the PM has developed over previous projects or in graduate school. The PM needs to work with a team consisting of a variety of people, each with an area of expertise in the applications that will be built and applied in the system. For instance, if the project were a clinical application for documentation, the build team would be separated into various smaller teams, such as a clinical documentation team composed primarily of nurses who had experience in documenting clinical notes. There would be a pharmacy team, medical team, and a list of other teams by department. These teams were brought together for the sole purpose of participating and assisting with the build of the system and then would go back to their clinical jobs after the EHR has been installed. This process could take anywhere from 6 to 9 months to 1.5 years depending on the size of the organization and installation. The five-step project management processes and concepts described previously represent some of the steps Amy would need to understand for both her graduate practicum and her new leadership role as manager.

WHAT IS PROJECT MANAGEMENT?

As discussed earlier, Amy told the CNO that she does not know what a project is but was reassured that many tasks are viewed as projects, be they large or small, such as the practicum project or Amy's sister's wedding. They all require some sort of organization or framework and management with a specific plan, due dates, start and end dates, and resources to be successful.

Undertaking Project Management: Examples

For many, the idea of project management is daunting. The concept of being a PM may be hard to comprehend, but actually taking on the role and being in charge is even more so. Understanding the basic concepts of PM, and defining and using metrics, the "who, what, why, how, when, and where" rule defined in Chapter 4, Planning: Project Management—Phase 2, when applying them can be simple, regardless of the size or purpose of the project. As long as the basic project management concepts and organizational methods are understood and applied, it does not matter who takes on project management: the APRN, DNP, CNO, or other healthcare professional, or those with other backgrounds, such as nursing faculty—as long as there is knowledge and there are PM skills. An APRN may encounter any or all of these management philosophies on a project. Nursing faculty have to plan courses, set due dates, and essentially manage each course and task as if it were a small project. To summarize, project management "is about knowing exactly what your goals are, how you're going to achieve them, what resources you'll need, and how long it will take you to reach that specific goal" (Paymo Academy, 2018, para. 1).

Constraints

Discussion, monitoring, and controlling barriers or constraints is a key function of the PM role. Constraints are limits, restrictions, and barriers to achieving the project goals and objectives. One of the most frequently discussed constraints is the ability to stay within the budget originally agreed to and developed with consultation and approval from the hospital's chief finance officer (CFO) and other key leadership. Managing the budget, schedule, quality, risk, and resources—those hired to work on the project— are responsibilities of the PM, just as they would be for any type of task. Amy will learn how to manage these items in her management course as she first learns to develop what is called the "scope document." The scope document discussed in Chapter 3, Design/Initiation: Project Management—Phase 1, is fundamental due to the need for a documented plan that defines specifics, such as when and how the plan will be carried out.

This type of plan also establishes boundaries of what will be done, how long it will take (time), how much it will cost, what resources/building supplies will be needed, and how many people it will take to get the work completed (resources) and what is not included. The three classic interdependencies—budget, schedule, and resources—which are critical to a project's success and are discussed further during the design phase (Chapter 3, Design/Initiation: Project Management—Phase 1) have now been updated to six or more constraints:

- Budget
- Schedule (time)
- Resources
- Risk
- Quality
- Scope (Shenoy, n.d.)

If one of these elements is out of plan, it will affect the other two, as will be discussed later.

PROJECT MANAGEMENT PROCESSES

Project management is a process of coordinating and directing team members to meet the formal, defined, approved goals and objectives outlined for the specific project. Managing a project will be accomplished using the skills developed in graduate school or from other projects, while also managing the constraints discussed previously to stay on time and on budget as you monitor quality as well as team and stakeholder satisfaction and performance. This is best accomplished when using consistent, standard processes in an organized way to meet the project goals and objectives. As mentioned, the standard processes used in project management are very similar to the steps in the nursing process. They include a list of activities or tasks that need to be completed in each of the five steps before the next step can be started:

- Design (initiation)
- Plan
- Apply/implement
- Regulate/monitor and control; supervise
- Conclude/close and evaluate

While the overall project phases are being supervised, all steps must also be regulated or controlled from the beginning. Although these five processes are the ones most frequently used, larger projects' processes may be broken into six or more components or phases so that the project can more easily be controlled. Some smaller projects include only four "official" phases as monitor and control are included in all stages, especially during the implementation. Regardless, all functions and processes must be included to prevent project failure and lead to a successful implementation. Organizing the project with specific, detailed steps adds a structure and a framework that are much easier to track and to change, if indicated.

REFLECTION QUESTIONS

1. What were some of the projects you have worked on before? How organized were they?
2. Were you able to complete them as expected by a certain due date?
3. Did you have a documented plan that you followed?

PRINCIPLES OF PROJECT MANAGEMENT

Basic principles and an understanding of project management are frequently acquired over a number of projects; learning what works well and where to focus key time and resources takes time and experience. Just as with any project, including the wedding previously discussed or Amy's master's practicum project, some of the first questions to ask during a critical analysis are:

- Why are we doing this project?
- Why do we need it? Who will benefit?
- Does it fit the organization's strategic mission and plan?
- What is the anticipated outcome or impact?

The APRN's role here is to help facilitate the discussions with end users who need the application in order to work effectively, information technologists, and other stakeholders. Additionally, if the APRN has assumed the role of the PM, it will be important to fully understand the five project management processes and how to apply them as listed previously.

Not only is it critical that the APRN in the role of PM be able to track, control, and closely monitor the five project management processes but to also understand other key responsibilities of project management, which are discussed in the following chapters. Those include regulating and controlling the project so that it is continually on time, on budget, and within scope of the project.

PROJECT MANAGEMENT: WHY DO WE NEED IT?

Historically, projects completed prior to 1950 were less organized, more chaotic, and haphazard than those undertaken today. According to Cleland and Ireland (2006), "it was [in] the 1950s, when project management was formally recognized as a distinct contribution arising from the [need for] management discipline" (pp. 1-4). Engineering was at the forefront of establishing project management. From the 1950s to today, the concept of project management has become a key management strategy in large corporations, such as IBM, Apple, and Microsoft, and now, more recently, in healthcare where there is a need to put more formalized structure and organization to tasks carried out in organizations. Nurses use an organized approach when providing care to patients. Patient care management requires an organizational framework—organizing processes similar to those used in project management are used to manage patient care.

Driving Forces Influencing Skills Development

Initially recommended in the Institute of Medicine report (IOM, 2011, 2013) and with the advent of the American Recovery and Reinvestment Act (ARRA) Initiative (2009), which contained the Health Information Technology for Economic and Clinical Health (HITECH) Act, came the mandate of what healthcare should do, including using EHRs to collect and monitor patient data, which further encouraged the use and development of technology by nurses, APRNs, and other healthcare professionals. The IOM report stresses that "nurses' roles, responsibilities and education should change to meet the needs of an aging, increasingly diverse population and to respond to a complex, evolving healthcare system. The recommendations in the report focus on the critical intersection between the health needs of patients across the lifespan and the readiness of the nursing workforce" (2013, para. 1). The Act's accompanying funding resources stimulated more rapid movement toward electronic data capture and health information exchanges (HIE; HealthIT.gov, n.d.). The HITECH Act is the portion of the ARRA that provides the U.S. Department of Health and Human Services (HHS) with the power to facilitate promotion and utilization of health information technology usage through government programs and Medicare and Medicaid, to levy fines if computer technology is not used in a meaningful way, and to collect and manage data in a way that will increase patient care efficiencies, improve care efficiencies using effective management strategies, such as monitor and control as well as evaluate, and cut healthcare dollars.

With the recommendations of the ARRA and accompanying mandates for hospitals to implement EHRs, there is an even greater need to implement standardized, organizing processes and methodologies to effectively and efficiently guide organizations through the many tasks needed to implement very complex EHRs in a very systematic way. Project management provides this standard process.

CRITICAL THINKING QUESTIONS AND ACTIVITIES

1. Why do you need to understand the steps of project management? Provide examples of a project using the foundation of project management.

2. What would happen if you did not have a project plan? How would you respond to a new manager who told you a plan is not needed?

3. You are planning a summer project. What are the five steps you need to plan and then develop the project? Where will you start—with the end date? Why, or why not?

4. What do you foresee as any barriers to starting your project?

SUMMARY

This introductory chapter was designed to provide an overview for Amy, the new manager and MSN student, of some of the project management skills that APRN, DNP, CNO, or other healthcare professionals need when undertaking the design, plan, implementation, and evaluation of a project.

Chapter 2, Advanced Practice Nurse Role Descriptions and Application of Project Management Concepts, discusses how well nurses and APRNs fit into the PM role as it models many of the same concepts used in the nursing process.

The project management standards originally developed in the 1950s by engineers were explained. Although based on proven concepts, this text was focused on defining concepts in a way that non-PMs, such as APRNs and other clinicians, will be better able to comprehend and apply to definitions and processes used on the business operations' side of a healthcare organization.

REFERENCES

American Association of Colleges of Nursing. (2014). *Expanded roles for advanced practice nurses.* Retrieved from http://www.aacn.nche.edu

American Nurses Association. (2008). *Nursing informatics: Scope and standards of practice.* Silver Spring, MD: Author.

American Nurses Association. (2010). *Nursing: Scope and standards of practice* (2nd ed.). Silver Spring, MD: Author.

American Nurses Association. (2015). *Nursing: Scope and standards of practice* (2nd ed.). Silver Spring, MD: Author.

American Organization of Nurse Executives. (2015). *AONE nurse executive competencies.* Chicago, IL: Author. Retrieved from https://www.aonl.org/sites/default/files/aone/nurse-executive-competencies.pdf

American Recovery and Reinvestment Act (ARRA) Initiative, HITECH Act. (2009). HealthIT.gov. Retrieved from https://www.hhs.gov/hipaa/for-professionals/special-topics/hitech-act-enforcement-interim-final-rule/index.html

Cleland, D., & Ireland, L. (2006). The evolution of project managment. In D. Cleland & R. Gareis (Eds.), *Global project management handbook* (2nd ed., pp. 1-3–1-19). New York, NY: McGraw-Hill Professional.

HealthIT.gov. (n.d.). *Health information exchange.* Retrieved from https://www.healthit.gov/topic/health-it-basics/health-information-exchange

Institute of Medicine. (2011). *The future of nursing: Leading change, advancing health.* Washington, DC: National Academies Press.

Institute of Medicine. (2013). The future of nursing IOM report. Retrieved from https://campaignforaction.org/resource/future-nursing-iom-report

Paymo Academy. (2018). *What is project management?* Retrieved from https://www.paymoapp.com/academy/what-is-project-management

Shenoy, S. (n.d.). *The 6 project constraints.* Retrieved from https://www.workfront.com/blog/the-6-project-constraints

Sipes, C. (2019). *Project management for the advanced practice nurse* (2nd ed.). New York, NY: Springer Publishing Company.

CHAPTER 2

ADVANCED PRACTICE NURSE ROLE DESCRIPTIONS AND APPLICATION OF PROJECT MANAGEMENT CONCEPTS

CAROLYN SIPES | SUSAN WALTZ

LEARNING OBJECTIVES

Upon completion of this chapter, the reader will be able to:

1. Discuss the correlation between the nursing process and project management.
2. List three roles that an advanced practice registered nurse (APRN) can assume.
3. Differentiate between information and computer literacy.
4. Discuss the value of establishing a framework for a project.
5. List two goals of using a standard process when designing a project.
6. Discuss theories that apply to project management.

OUTLINE

- Key Terms
- Introduction

- History and Driving Forces to Develop Skills for the Role of the APRN
- Foundational Project Management Theories That Support Decision Making
- Correlation Between the Nursing Process and Project Management
- Understanding the Differences Between Information and Computer Literacy: Why Is This Important?
- APRN, DNP, Nurse Executive, and Leadership Essential Skills
- Nurse Leadership Roles and Essential Skills
- Other Advanced Practice Nurse Roles
- Competency Assessment
- Summary

KEY TERMS

- Competencies
- Computer literacy
- Doctor of nursing practice (DNP)
- Health Information Technology for Economic and Clinical Health Act (HITECH)
- Institute of Medicine (IOM)
- Informatics nurse specialist (INS)
- Information literacy
- Nurse informaticist (NI)
- Nursing process

INTRODUCTION

The focus of this chapter is to help nurses understand the value, skills, and knowledge they will develop when reviewing applicable theories and learning the principles of project management that have very similar concepts as in the nursing process and that are applied by an APRN in practice. Not only are the steps that are used to manage patient care required in practice, but nurses are expected to possess the skills, knowledge, and ability to apply concepts of project management in today's practice (Project Management Institute [PMI], 2013). The American Nurses Association (ANA, 2015) and Foster and Sethares (2017) emphasize that "informatics competencies are needed by all nurses whether or not they specialize in informatics. As nurse settings become more ubiquitous computing environments, all nurses must be both information and computer literate" (p. 1). The methodology and technology used in informatics are part of project management in that the knowledge, techniques, and competencies required and developed using informatics help APRNs to better manage their practice.

> **QUESTIONS TO CONSIDER BEFORE READING ON**
>
> 1. Discuss project management skills needed for any project.
> 2. What are some of the project management skills identified by the Office of the National Coordinator for Health Information Technology that are required of EHR users?
> 3. Why is there a gap in APRNs who function as project managers (PMs)?
> 4. Why are theories important to project management?
> 5. Discuss four key theories that guide a project.

HISTORY AND DRIVING FORCES TO DEVELOP SKILLS FOR THE ROLE OF THE APRN

A brief discussion of driving forces is provided in Chapter 1, Basic Project Management for Advanced Practice Nurses and Healthcare Professionals, but the major driving forces for nurses to advance their skills and practice levels are listed in the Institute of Medicine (IOM) report (2011, 2012) *The Future of Nursing: Leading Change, Advancing Health Through Better Data Collection and Improved Information Infrastructure.* This report sets forth a mandate and challenge to the practice of nursing; it suggests the need to transform the nursing profession as well as the healthcare system as a whole. In this significant report, there are eight core recommendations.

Of these, the ones most significant to nurses developing skills and competencies in project management are listed as follows:

1. Expand opportunities for nurses to lead and diffuse collaborative improvement efforts.

2. Ensure that nurses engage in lifelong learning, such as continuing toward a doctor of nursing practice (DNP).

3. Prepare and enable nurses to lead change to advance health.

4. Build an infrastructure for the collection and analysis of inter-professional healthcare workforce data.

Historically, in 2004 President George W. Bush outlined a plan to ensure that most Americans have an electronic health record (EHR) by 2014 and stated that "[b]y computerizing health records, we can avoid dangerous medical mistakes, reduce costs, and improve care" (Bush, 2004, para. 54). Then in 2009, the Health Information Technology for Economic and Clinical Health Act (HITECH), enacted as part of the American Recovery and Reinvestment Act of 2009, advanced incentives for providers to become meaningful users of EHRs (American Recovery and Reinvestment Act [ARRA] Initiative, 2014). To be competent as an EHR user requires knowledge and competency in project management and informatics, specifically data entry, analysis, facilitation between information technology (IT) and clinicians, workflow design, management of projects and resources, and, most importantly, change management (Office of the National Coordinator for Health Information Technology, 2014).

The push to change the healthcare system to improve patient quality, safety, and outcomes, through effective development and implementation of EHRs, has led to an increase in demand for project management skills. Project management is especially suited to APRNs as health systems realize they need to update legacy, older systems in order to be more efficient when developing and managing patients' medical and health records. A critical point overlooked in all of these mandates from national organizations was the fact that very few in the workforce were competent or possessed the skills needed to implement any of the recommendations without extensive training. A report by the Health Resources and Services Administration (HRSA) suggested that the implementation of an EHR system requires skills in leadership and management of a project team that few possess (U.S. Department of Health and Human Services [HHS], 2014). Skill requirements are further supported by Provost (2018) in a number of articles describing the needs to provide for quality improvement in healthcare, including an article that defines the five principles needed in order to move the process of quality improvement forward. (See "Quality Improvement in Healthcare: 5 Guiding Principles" [Provost, 2018].) It is also important to understand basic theories related to project management as foundational guides for the discipline. These are discussed later in this chapter.

A partial list of additional project management skills needed to undertake any project, large or small, to keep it well organized and managed, also includes:

- Good communication skills and processes—both verbal and written
- Steps in the implementation process require close monitoring to stay on time and on budget
- Risk management; risks need to be defined, documented, tracked, and mitigated
- Monitoring resources
- Controlling quality

This list requires a skill mix of project management, computer literacy, and informatics. Finally, it should be noted that the following skills and knowledge are needed in any management position or other leadership roles, not just project management:

- Ability to successfully create and implement a plan
- Demonstrate ability to organize
- Ability to document processes and apply tracking tools
- Ability to conduct accurate assessments and identify gaps in processes
- Understand and successfully apply concepts of change management
- Ability to create effective, concise status, executive, and other reports and conduct meetings
- Understanding of foundational theories to support decision making

Other roles and skills that APRNs might assume are also discussed later. Some of the information included was retrieved from job websites in a search for specific, updated roles and skills required today.

In the past, the leaders and committees who developed then set forth mandates outlined as driving forces further identified tasks and skills needed to move healthcare reform forward. But many times when organizations tried to hire someone with the skills needed for the job, such as managing an EHR implementation, they found a gap in both the skill levels and education of APRNs with regard to knowledge and management skills. APRNs are proficient in assessing and providing patient care but lack the management skills needed to plan and organize a clinic, manage resources, budgets, time, and many other aspects of project management.

FOUNDATIONAL PROJECT MANAGEMENT THEORIES THAT SUPPORT DECISION MAKING

Theory shapes practice and provides a method for expressing key ideas regarding the principles of nursing practice (Walker & Avant, 2011). Nursing theory is developed from groups of concepts and describes their interrelationships, thus presenting a systematic view of nursing-related events. The purpose of theory is to describe, explain, predict, and/or prescribe (Chinn & Kramer, 2011; Reed & Shearer, 2013; Risjord, 2009; Walker & Avant, 2011). Regardless of the theory level, it is important for *all* nurses to understand nursing theories as they provide the foundation for practice (Sipes, 2016). The theories identified in the following sections include a partial list of those that contribute to supporting the framework and decision-making constructs of project management. This list is an overview; detailed content can be found when exploring each theory further, but full content is not included here.

Data–Information–Knowledge–Wisdom (DIKW) Framework

The initial model evaluated for use in NI was the DIKW framework, which originated from the computer informatics and information sciences, particularly knowledge management (Blum, 1986). The ANA describes "wisdom" as the ability to evaluate information and knowledge within the context of caring and use judgment to make care decisions (ANA, 2008; Matney, Brewster, Sward, Cloyes, & Staggers, 2011). The DIKW model has been valuable in advancing the independent field of NI by providing a framework for what data are and how data are applied (Matney, Avant, & Staggers, 2015; Ronquillo, Currie, & Rodney, 2016).

Benner: Novice-to-Expert Model

In 1989, Dreyfus and Dreyfus (1980) created the Dreyfus model, which suggests that in the acquisition and development of a skill, one passes through four levels of proficiency—novice, advanced beginner, competent, proficient—to become an expert. Benner (1982, 2004) adapted the model to explain how nursing students and professional nurses acquire nursing skills, including NI.

Chaos Theory

Chaos theory is associated with the butterfly effect, a theory that states that a small change can result in a significant effect later. Chaos theory deals with differences in outcomes that depend on the conditions present at the starting point. If you have been involved in the implementation of a new EHR at a healthcare facility, you might have seen how the plan in place at the beginning of the process changed and did not result in the original planned outcome in the end—the plan changed overtime.

General Systems Theory

In systems theory the focus is on the interaction among the various parts of the system instead of recognizing each individual part, considering the whole greater than the sum of its parts (Current Nursing, 2012; von Bertalanffy, 1968).

Cognitive Science

Cognitive science provides the framework for designing tools to support computer and screen development, for example, understanding the steps for constructive use of information and information processing to gain knowledge (Staggers & Thompson, 2002).

Computer Science

Computer science is the study of algorithms used to solve computation problems by using the computer as the tool that defines and connects the steps in a process.

Change Theory

One of the most frequently used theories is Lewin's change theory, which provides a framework for managing change, most frequently seen with changes that come with the implementation of an EHR. It has three stages—unfreezing, change, and refreezing—as well as three major concepts: driving forces, restraining forces, and equilibrium (Barrow & Toney-Butler, 2019; Kaminski, 2011).

Diffusion of Innovation Theory

Rogers's diffusion of innovation theory explores leaders, followers, and how the media can influence opinion leaders and followers. According to Mohammadi, Poursaberi, and Salahshoor (2018), personal characteristics influence whether people adopt an innovation rapidly.

Implementation Science

Implementation science involves increased use of theoretical approaches to provide better understanding and explanation of how and why an implementation succeeds or fails. Theoretical approaches used in implementation science have three overarching aims: describing and/or guiding the process of translating research into practice (process models); understanding and/or explaining what influences implementation outcomes (determinant frameworks, classic theories, and implementation theories); and evaluating implementation (evaluation frameworks; Nilsen, 2015).

The theories just identified are those used by various organizations as they begin to implement a new project with the realization that foundational concepts and frameworks can lead to a successful outcome.

CORRELATION BETWEEN THE NURSING PROCESS AND PROJECT MANAGEMENT

Although the concept of project management seems foreign to many, there is a common thread that applies to the different types of work nurses do (i.e., the nursing process—one of the first core principles of nursing practice nurses learn to apply when delivering the best evidence-based patient care). Suggestions that nurses will understand and be able to apply the five basic principles of project management arise from project management's similarity to the five steps of the nursing process. The steps and phases are similar to some project management terms and tasks, but differences may be only an issue of semantics. Ultimately, nurses, especially as they achieve more advanced levels in their practice, will find many similarities between processes of project management and the nursing process. The main difference is they are working with a project instead of patients (Table 2.1).

TABLE 2.1 Correlation of the Nursing Process to Project Management Concepts

NURSING PROCESS	PROJECT MANAGEMENT
1. Assessment—collect and analyze patient data 2. Diagnosis; develop precare plan 3. Outcomes plan; goal development 4. Implement care plan 5. Evaluate plan; update plan	1. Design/initiate project—current state workflow analysis; gap analysis 2. Develop project plan 3. Implement project plan 4. Monitor and control project 5. Close project; evaluate lessons learned

SOURCE: Sipes, C. (2016). *Project management for the advance practice nurse* (p. 19). New York, NY: Springer Publishing Company.

In summary, just as the nursing process provides an organizing framework for patient care management, the project management processes provide the organizational framework for a project or other roles where an organizing framework would be useful (Figures 2.1 and 2.2).

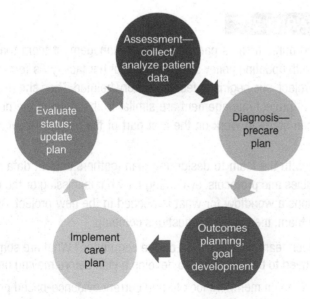

FIGURE 2.1 The five steps of the nursing process.

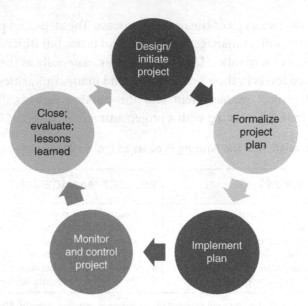

FIGURE 2.2 The five phases of project management.

SOURCE: Sipes, C. (2016). *Project management for the advance practice nurse* (p. 19). New York, NY: Springer Publishing Company.

CASE SCENARIO 2.1

Terry, registered nurse (RN), is part of a project management team that has been charged with updating policy and protocols for her facility. As Terry looks at the overall project, she begins to feel a bit overwhelmed. Then she remembers the steps of project management are similar to the steps of the nursing process and then starts to work on the first part of the project—developing a plan.

Terry works with the team to design the plan (gathers current data about the current policies and protocols, evaluating for what is missing or the gaps) and then develops a workflow for what is needed in the new project. As she works with the team, the following questions come up:

1. How can each team member work on the committee? What are some tasks that need to be completed to develop a plan before moving on?

2. Where would team members look to find current evidence-based practices (EBP) to support new policies?

(continued)

During this planning step, each person begins conducting research to find current EBP to support the selected protocols and policies. At this point, more questions come up:

1. Is the team computer literate? Will they be able to successfully conduct research?
2. What can be done to help the team become more computer literate?

> ► **QUESTIONS TO CONSIDER**
> **BEFORE READING ON**
>
> Discuss the differences between computer and information literacy.
> 1. What roles might the APRN and DNP assume?
> 2. What are some of the basic requirements in today's practice?
> 3. How has healthcare changed in that the roles' requirements have changed as well?

UNDERSTANDING THE DIFFERENCES BETWEEN INFORMATION AND COMPUTER LITERACY: WHY IS THIS IMPORTANT?

As APRNs develop more advanced leadership and management skills, they must also become more information and computer literate. As noted earlier, the ANA statement emphasizes that "informatics competencies are needed by all nurses whether or not they specialize in informatics. As nurse settings become more ubiquitous computing environments, all nurses must be both information and computer literate" (ANA, 2008, p. 2).

It is important to understand the differences between information and computer literacy because they are required today as part of demonstrated competency in information management, which includes applying the concepts and framework of project management (PMI, 2013). There are several definitions of computer literacy. A basic definition is as follows: "Computer literacy is the knowledge and ability to use computers and related technology efficiently, understand computer concepts and limitations, and possess a range of skills covering levels from elementary use to programming and advanced problem solving" (ANA, 2015, p. 28).

In addition to computer literacy, understanding the concepts of information literacy is essential to developing skills needed by the APRN, especially as nursing today is becoming more high-tech (ANA, 2015).

The beginning of the 21st century has been called the Information Age because of the explosion of information output and information sources. Information literacy forms the basis for lifelong learning. It is common to all disciplines, to all learning environments, and to all levels of education. It enables learners to master content and extend their investigations, become more self-directed, and assume greater control over their own learning. Information literacy is the set of skills needed to understand, find, retrieve, analyze, and use information (Association of College and Research Libraries, 2014, p. 1).

"Computer literacy is a core competency needed in health care, and should be taught in nursing curricula at all levels. In addition, information literacy must be integrated into practice and used to support knowledge management. These are the foundations of informatics competencies" (ANA, 2015, p. 28). To be considered literate in computers, an APRN should have experience and competencies when using computers and applications as well as understand some of the basic techniques needed in order to support other nurses and peers. Again, as mentioned earlier, the APRN employs principles of both informatics and project management to be considered competent and literate in computers and IT. As indicated, many comparisons have been made between the five steps of the nursing process and project management. As noted by Research Gate (2014), nurses are well suited for IT implementations that follow the nursing process of assessment, diagnosis, planning, implementation, and evaluation.

The American Association of Colleges of Nursing (AACN, 2008, 2011) defined essential and expected competencies for nursing informatics education and graduation that apply to developing project management skills. The competencies expected for graduation are defined at three levels: those required for bachelor of science in nursing (BSN), master of science in nursing (MSN), and DNP. For example, competencies expected at the DNP level for graduation include the ability to design, select, evaluate, and use processes; to analyze and communicate critical elements; to develop and execute plans; and to demonstrate leadership (Fulton, Meek, & Walker, 2014). All of these competencies are the same as those expected from a PM.

Informatics and electronic health/medical records are being mandated by federal mandates with professional organizations encouraging the adoption of such electronic records in clinical practice. Health information record systems are now functional systems through which nurses navigate technology, documents, and plan patient care (Foster & Sethares, 2017; Gardner & Jones, 2012, p. 1702). Because of the rapidly evolving changes in health information requirements and technology, there is also a need for nurses to acquire higher level computer and information competencies that are part of project management. As discussed in an article by Abu Raddaha (2017), "[n]urses should be able to demonstrate basic nursing informatics competencies when dealing with computers and software applications used in healthcare settings" (p. 32). Consider if you are the PM but do not have computer skills—what would you do? All these tie together in the need for basic skills and understanding to be effective in your roles.

The role of the PM is critical to the success of a project. Many times leadership may overlook the value of a PM with the misconception that another person in any leadership role can also assume the role while also completing other duties. It is important to note that the role of the PM is different and should be different from operations or other functional managers. The role of the APRN as a seasoned PM will bring skills and knowledge to the project, including a thorough understanding of the key concepts and principles of project management.

APRN, DNP, NURSE EXECUTIVE, AND LEADERSHIP ESSENTIAL SKILLS

This book defines the functional areas and competencies as well as the accountabilities and activities required in the role of a PM. Although this book is used primarily as a course text, resource, and guide, the basic concepts and processes in the book will help develop and guide skills and knowledge needed for other health informatics specialties as well as other healthcare providers, executives, and leaders who may be assuming a project management role in the healthcare industry as a number of project management competences are also standards of practice for nurse informaticists (NIs), such as standards 1 to 6 (ANA, 2015). This book is used by many who need to have organizing guidelines necessary to develop a project for a graduate practicum in a master's or doctoral program.

According to the ANA, the following competencies are essential for *all* beginning and practicing nurses:

- Basic computer literacy, including the ability to use basic desktop applications and electronic communication

■ The ability to use IT to support clinical and administrative processes, which presumes information literacy to support evidence-based practice

■ The ability to access data and perform documentation via computerized patient records

■ The ability to support patient safety initiatives via the use of IT (ANA, 2015)

As has been discussed, nurses even at the advanced level do not have the basic competencies needed for most nursing jobs today. More than ever, nursing has become and now is considered a high-tech discipline. For nurses entering an APRN program in graduate school, the project management framework is beneficial in courses where the goal of the course is to assess, develop, and design and then implement best practices for a project that might address a specific practice issue for a healthcare organization. Project management concepts are especially important when collaborating with others in nursing practice, nursing leadership, or other interdisciplinary fields of study or healthcare disciplines. Most nurses who enter into graduate school are unfamiliar with project management processes until they realize its correlation to the nursing process that they have used for many years. As they continue the career path through graduate school, they will develop and apply the organizational skills they have learned, but now it will be while designing and planning the framework they will use to develop a practicum project required for graduation and then in their practices after graduation, especially as a clinical manager.

Additionally, at this point in the graduate program, the APRN will need to evaluate competencies for basic computer skills as well as information and computer literacy described here (HIMSS, 2017). These skills will have to be assessed prior to taking on the role of a PM, or other management roles, as they are now considered a basic requirement to function well in those roles.

▶ **QUESTIONS TO CONSIDER BEFORE READING ON**

1. What are some roles of a nurse administrator, nurse executive, chief nursing informatics officer (CNIO)?

2. What are some of the competencies required of nurse leaders?

3. How do these roles differ from project management?

NURSE LEADERSHIP ROLES AND ESSENTIAL SKILLS

The ANA (2016), AONE (2015), and American Nurses Credentialing Center (ANCC, n.d.) education requirements and skills outline core abilities necessary for the nurse administrator, nurse executive, and CNIO. In all of the competencies listed, you will see overlap in many of these as they are also project management and nursing informatics competencies— they are not mutually exclusive to one specialty. These include:

- Accountability and advocacy for employees
- Clinical care delivery and optimal patient outcomes
- Ability and experience to use management skills
- Ability to embrace change and innovations to manage resources effectively
- Ability to negotiate and resolve conflict
- Ability to communicate effectively
- Collaborate in nursing research and translate evidence into practice and collaborate to investigate care delivery models across the continuum
- Safety, quality, and risk management
- Strategic, financial, and human resource management
- Assess the effectiveness of delivery models, develop new delivery models, and participate in the design of facilities

The Nurse Administrator

The nurse administrator is a "registered nurse whose primary responsibility is to manage health care delivery services ... in a variety of settings ... and must be prepared ... in such fields as information management and evidence-based care and management" (ANA, 2016, p. 6). The nurse administrator competencies include those listed previously and many of those listed in the nurse executive competencies. The competency requirements depend on the organization.

The Nurse Executive

As a nurse executive, the requirement is to develop and implement evaluation of six board standards for nurse administrators and executives, including assessment, diagnosis of problems, and identification of outcomes, planning, implementation, and evaluation as well as other organizational responsibilities. Evidence-based management is an important process that should be implemented in healthcare because the work environment in healthcare experiences greater turbulence, chaos, and instability than it does in other disciplines. Untested and dated management practices are no longer useful and may even be detrimental to patient care. Roles that use the standards of practice and are evidence based are discussed, although the specific content and expectations within a project will depend on the specialty area and components required in the project; however, the basic principles and processes are the same for any project that might be developed. According to the American Organization of Nurse Executives (AONE), competencies require that there should be abilities to do the following:

- Use data and other sources of evidence to inform decision making; use evidence for establishment of standards, practices, and patient care models in the organization.
- Design and interpret outcome measures.
- Articulate the organization's performance improvement program and goals by establishing quality metrics using measurable goals; identify the problem/process.
- Analyze root causes or variations from quality standards, improve processes and apply EBP, and control solutions and sustain success.
- Identify areas of risk/liability, facilitate staff education on risk management and compliance issues, develop systems that result in prompt reporting of potential liability for areas of projects, identify early warning predictability indications for errors, and correct areas of potential liability.
- Use knowledge of classic and contemporary systems thinking in problem solving and decision making, model systems thinking as an expectation of leaders and staff, and consider the impact of nursing decisions on the healthcare organization as a whole.
- Adapt leadership style to situation needs, use change theory to implement change, and serve as a change leader.
- Uphold ethical principles and corporate compliance standards.
- Develop and manage project budgets and expenditures, manage financial resources, and participate in the negotiation and monitoring of contracts.

- Involve nurses and other staff in decisions that affect their practice.

- Create the operational objectives, goals, and specific strategies required to achieve the strategic outcome; conduct SWOT and gap analyses; defend the business case; utilize the balanced scorecard analysis to manage change; and evaluate achievement of operational objectives and goals.

- Use technology to support improvement of clinical and financial performance; collaborate to prioritize for the establishment of IT resources; participate in evaluation of enabling technology in practice settings; use data management systems for decision making; identify technological trends, issues, and new developments as they apply to patient care; demonstrate skills in assessing data integrity and quality; and provide leadership for the adoption and implementation of information systems (AONE, 2015, pp. 4–8).

CNIO

If the APRN were to assume a job as a CNIO, the skills and expectations would include (per the HIMSS website's job description) the ability to do the following:

- Lead the region in the strategy, development, and implementation of IT to support nursing, nursing practice, and clinical applications, by collaborating with area chief nursing officers (CNOs) on the clinical and administrative decision-making process

- Develop clinical systems strategy by collaborating with the regional chief medical information officer (CMIO)

- Optimize the use of existing clinical systems for nurses, physicians, and other multidisciplinary care providers by attending to their information management needs

- Practice an executive nature comprising complex leadership and administrative components, associated with critical healthcare issues and activities that influence the organizational mission, healthcare, and policy

- Collaborate with other executives for strategic planning, decision making, and problem solving, as well as developing resource utilization strategies to improve organizational performance

- Use project management experience to advance projects (HIMSS, 2014)

This section included specific correlations to both project management and nurse leadership skills and competency requirements where you can see considerable overlap. The following sections include descriptions of other specialty areas for the advanced practice nurse and some of the competencies and skills that might be required in those specialty areas.

CASE SCENARIO 2.1 (continued)

Terry, RN, is beginning to learn the process and steps required to work as part of the project team. She has a number of questions regarding the different requirements of others who will be working on the team and what their contributions to the team could be. She understands there will be a nurse practitioner and clinical nurse specialist (CNS) as part of the team.

1. What are some basic skills they will bring to the team?

2. What will their roles be—in addition to the PM—or will one of them be the PM and lead the team?

> **QUESTIONS TO CONSIDER BEFORE READING ON**
> 1. What are four advanced practice roles?
> 2. Discuss the competencies and skills required for each role.
> 3. How do these roles differ from the project management role?

OTHER ADVANCED PRACTICE NURSE ROLES

The Association of periOperative Registered Nurses (AORN) defines an APRN as a nurse practitioner (NP), CNS, certified registered nurse anesthetist (CRNA), or certified nurse-midwife (CNM). The National Council of State Boards of Nursing (NCSBN) and others define an advanced practice nurse (APRN) as an RN with the expert knowledge, complex decision-making skills, and clinical competencies necessary for expanded practice. This differentiates APRNs from RNs in that they are capable of taking on more complex casework and handling those cases with greater independence and discretion. Some of the job functions and skills necessary for an APRN listed by AORN are that the APRN should be able to do the following:

- Direct patient care
- Provide consultation for nursing staff by implementing improvements in healthcare delivery systems
- Assess, plan, implement, evaluate, and document care (project management skills)

The manager roles require that the APRN be experienced in staffing, budgeting, and resource management—all project management skills.

- Manage staff, such as certified nursing assistants, RNs, licensed practical nurses, surgical technologists, and other allied healthcare providers; schedule staff; hire and fire staff; and mentor staff (resource management)
- Maintain department or unit's budget (budgeting)
- Communicate organizational issues to the staff (communication)
- Oversee daily activities within their department or unit (project management)
- Collaborate with other departments and physicians on departmental issues

At the director level, AORN requires that the APRN skills include, but are not limited to, responsibility for the operation of the department and for the measurement, assessment, and continuous improvement of the department's performance (Medscape, 2014).

The NP and CNS

NPs and CNSs prepared at the master's or doctoral level perform advanced practice nursing in an assigned specialty population throughout the continuum of care. The CNS serves in all three spheres of influence: complex patient care and research, systems processes and policies, and staff development and nursing practice. The CNS influences patient- and family-centered care and evidence-based nursing practice, promotes best practices for the interprofessional patient care team, and promotes evidence-based organizational change to meet the needs of the assigned population. This CNS is responsible for the development, implementation, promotion, and day-to-day coordination of this program. Skills also include leading groups and implementing change, as well as the ability to respond to and manage change. The CNS must have the ability to communicate effectively both orally and in writing, manage multiple simultaneous tasks and prioritize appropriately, as well as have knowledge of dynamics of group process (Clinical Nurse Specialist, 2018).

Many times, NPs and CNSs manage and own their own practices. They also achieve a higher level of education, the DNP.

The NI

The NI differentiates from other informatics specialties, such as medicine, pharmacy, and dentistry, where the focus is more on database management. Each informatics specialty is aligned uniquely with its primary role, requiring that informatics nurse specialists (INSs) augment their base of nursing knowledge with unique informatics skills. In the past, the definition of the NI focused solely on data collection and the use of data; many organizations still are not choosing to implement the use of an NI until post–electronic medical record (EMR) implementation (when electronic data are robust). According to the ANA, in 2008, the beginning nurse focused primarily on developing and using skills that rely on the ability to retrieve and enter data in an electronic format that is relevant to patient care, the analysis and interpretation of information as part of planning care, the use of informatics applications designed for nursing practice, and the implementation of policies relevant to information (ANA, 2015). According to the HIMSS (2018) statement regarding NI functions, the NI has advanced from a discipline previously focused on EMR implementation to one that ultimately facilitates and optimizes technology and informatics tools that help clinicians provide better care and positive health outcomes for patients as they monitor the outcomes. Additionally, it is important to note that the NI role is rapidly evolving in the functional areas and now plays a more integral role in the early planning phases of system development and management. This is why the NI and INS need to develop project management skills.

The INS

The INS is often responsible for implementing or coordinating projects involving multiple disciplines. The INS is expected to interact with professionals involved in all phases of the information systems life cycle and with professionals in all aspects of system utilization. "Both the INS and NI support consumers, patients, nurses, and other providers in their decision making in all roles and settings. This support is accomplished through the use of information structures, information process and information technology" (ANA, 2015, p. 1). ANA (2008) defines the level 3 nurse as an INS who is an RN with advanced preparation and knowledge in information management. A partial list of skills includes the ability to incorporate critical thinking, process skills, data management skills, project management and systems development life cycle skills, and computer skills into areas of nursing practice. Some of the more advanced competencies that the INS will have include:

- Proficiency with informatics applications to support all areas of nursing practice, including project management, quality-improvement activities, and research, as well as system design, development, analysis, implementation, support, maintenance, and evaluation—all skills that a PM possesses

- Fiscal management

- Skills in critical thinking, data management and processing, decision making, system development, and computer skills

- Identification and provision of data for decision making (ANA, 2008)

An INS in the role of administrator and leader would potentially work as a CNIO (HIMSS, 2014). In a midlevel management role, the INS's activities might include conducting "a needs analysis, design, development, evaluation, and implementation" of a system (ANA, 2008, p. 18). This is an area that would require project management skills.

DNP Practice

The DNP graduate's practice includes not only direct care but also a focus on the needs of patients, a target population, a set of populations, or a broad community. The DNP (Zaccagnini & White, 2017):

- Must be able to conceptualize new care delivery models that are based in contemporary nursing science and that are feasible within current organizational, political, cultural, and economic perspectives

- Must be skilled in working within organizational and policy arenas and in the actual provision of patient care alone and/or with others
- Must understand principles of practice management, including conceptual and practical strategies for balancing productivity with quality of care
- Must be able to assess the impact of practice policies and procedures on meeting the health needs of the patient populations with whom he or she practices
- Must be proficient in quality-improvement strategies and in creating and sustaining changes at the organizational and policy levels
- Must be able to manage corresponding change management in organizational arrangements, manage organizational and professional cultures, and manage the financial structures necessary to support practice
- Must be able to evaluate the cost-effectiveness of care and use principles of economics and finance to redesign effective and realistic care delivery strategies
- Must be able to organize care to address emerging practice problems and the ethical dilemmas that emerge as new diagnostic and therapeutic technologies evolve
- Must be able to assess risk and collaborate with others to manage risks ethically, based on professional standards
- Must be able to design, select, and use information systems/ technology to evaluate programs of care, outcomes of care, and care systems; using information systems/technology, the DNP must be able to apply budget and productivity tools, practice information systems and decision supports, and use web-based learning or intervention tools to support decision making and manage and provide leadership

To summarize, skills needed by any or all of the advanced practice roles defined include:

- Organization skills and management skills
- Clinical reengineering—workflow and gap analysis
- Change management

- Work processes' support
- Information management
- Time management
- Resource management
- Leadership
- Communication skills
- Strategic planning
- Decision making and decision support
- Problem solving
- Budget development and cost monitoring

All of the skills listed, and others, are required of a PM. During the initial design and planning phase of the project, the APRN will be expected to have skill and experience in developing the management and budget tools that will be needed to track the various project functions.

Further, because roles are frequently confused with position titles and with the lack of standardization in the new specialty of nursing informatics, the ANA has provided a description of some of the functional areas for INSs and NIs that are still relevant and are evolving today. These include:

- Administration, leadership, and management
- Analysis
- Compliance and integrity management
- Consultation
- Coordination, facilitation, and integration
- Development
- Educational and professional development
- Policy development and advocacy
- Research and evaluation (ANA, 2008, pp. 17–18)

The expanded use of health information technology (HIT) promotes interprofessional development and collaboration as well as patient involvement in the utilization of healthcare devices. This will require the APRN to address all environments and all levels of user ability to accommodate the various devices being developed (Table 2.2).

TABLE 2.2 Partial List of Essential Roles and Skills of an APRN

AS CHANGE AGENTS	An inherent function of the APRN is that of a change agent, involving collaboration and consultation with other healthcare providers (AACN)
AS LEADERS	Have excellent communication skills, conduct risk assessment, coalition building with business acumen, and have strategic application knowledge
ARE COMFORTABLE WITH CHANGE AND COMPLEXITY IN DYNAMIC ENVIRONMENTS	The use of evidence-based practice necessitates the implementation of change, with the APRN as change agent (Medscape, 2014)
ABLE TO GUIDE AND CULTIVATE PEOPLE SKILLS	Guides others in the development of effective oral and written communication skills, including communication with project stakeholders (www.healthsystem.virginia.edu)
HAVE A BROAD AND FLEXIBLE TOOLKIT OF TECHNIQUES	Adapt approach to the context and constraints of each project, knowing that no "one size" can fit all the varieties of projects
HAVE THE KNOWLEDGE TO DEVELOP AND UTILIZE A VARIETY OF TOOLS	Utilize the tools to track the project progress from start to completion
TAKE OWNERSHIP FOR THE PROJECT	Assume responsibility and accountability for the project

APRN, advanced practice registered nurse.

SOURCE: Adapted from American Association of Colleges of Nursing. (2011). *The essentials of master's education in nursing* (pp. 5–29). Retrieved from https://www.aacnnursing.org/Portals/42/Publications/MastersEssentials11.pdf

Although the survey referred to in Table 2.3 was completed by HIMSS for NIs, the directive for all nurses to have skills in project management has been recognized and recommended by such organizations as ANA, ANCC, and the Quality and Safety Education for Nurses (QSEN) survey funded by the Robert Wood Johnson Foundation (RWJF). The table lists results from the NI workforce survey of the top five job responsibilities. The original survey was conducted by the HIMSS in 2011 and updated in 2017. The emphasis on collecting these data was to demonstrate that the NIs and INSs should be employed earlier rather than later with an EHR system implementation. This survey provides evidence that NIs and INSs should be employed not only after data collection but also during the first decision-making processes.

TABLE 2.3 HIMSS NI Workforce Survey's Top Five Job Responsibilities—Application to APRNs

#1 Systems implementation; utilization/optimization #2 Systems development #3 Quality initiatives #4 Liaison with IT and other clinicians #5 Strategic planning

SOURCE: Data from Healthcare Information and Management Systems Society. (2017). *2017 nursing informatics workforce survey.* Retrieved from https://www.himss.org/ni-workforce -survey

COMPETENCY ASSESSMENT

Today many colleges, universities, and national organizations require that all nurses complete a competency assessment that provides feedback regarding the level of skills the nurse has and the skills needed in order to achieve a particular skill level. Employers rely more heavily on national organizations and universities to provide the necessary education and certifications the nurse will need for a specific job.

Now there is more information in the literature on how to self-assess nursing informatics competencies.

The partial list includes:

- Hunter, K., McGonigle, D., Hebda, T., Sipes, C., Hill, T., & Lamblin, J. (2015). TIGER-based assessment of nursing informatics competencies (TANIC). In A. Rocha, A. Correia, S. Costanzo, & L. Reis (Eds.), *New contributions in information systems and technologies. Advances in intelligent systems and computing* (Vol. 353). Cham, Switzerland: Springer. doi:10.1007/978-3-319-16486-1_17

- Sipes, C., Hunter, K., McGonigle, D., Hebda, T., Hill, T., & Lamblin, J. (2016). Competency skills assessment: Successes and areas for improvement identified during collaboration between informaticists and a national organization. *Studies in Health Technology and Informatics: Nursing Informatics 2016, 225,* 43–47. doi:10.3233/978-1-61499-658-3-43

- Sipes, C., McGonigle, D., Hunter, K., Hebda, T., Hill, T., & Lamblin, J. (2016). Operationalizing the TANIC and NICA-L3/L4 tools to improve informatics competencies. *Studies in Health Technology and Informatics: Nursing Informatics 2016, 225,* 292–296. doi:10.3233/978-1-61499-658-3-292

■ Sipes, C. (2016). Project management: Essential skill of nurse informaticists. *Studies in Health Technology and Informatics: Nursing Informatics 2016, 225*, 252–256. doi:10.3233/978-1-61499-658-3-252

■ Hill, T., McGonigle, D., Hunter, K., Sipes, C., & Hebda, T. (2014). An instrument for assessing advanced nursing informatics competencies. *Journal of Nursing Education and Practice, 4*(7), 104–112. doi:10.5430/jnep.v4n7p104

■ Hunter, K., McGonigle, D., Hill, T., Hebda, T., & Sipes, C. (2014). Self-reported assessment of basic and informatics specialist/innovator nursing informatics competencies: TANIC© and NICA L3/L4©. *Nursing Informatics Today, 29*(2), 4–6.

■ Hunter, K., McGonigle, D., & Hebda, T. (2013). The integration of informatics content in baccalaureate and graduate nursing education: A status report. *Nurse Educator, 38*(3), 110–113. doi:10.1097/NNE.0b013e31828dc292

■ McGonigle, D., Hunter, K., Sipes, C., & Hebda, T. (2014). Why nurses need to understand nursing informatics. *AORN Journal, 100*(3), 324–327. doi:10.1016/j.aorn.2014.06.012

CRITICAL THINKING QUESTIONS AND ACTIVITIES

You are a new INS, just passed your certification exam and now looking for a leadership role as an advanced practice nurse in informatics. You know that NI and INS roles have evolved so that essential skills and competencies have changed considerably requiring more leadership skills over the past 3 years—it is no longer as much about data collection but requires much wider responsibility now.

1. How would you start your job search?

2. Which websites would you use to find a job that now meets your skill set?

3. Which nursing informatics organizations would you use to network with?

Make a list of your competencies and what you would like to do—would it be working with others in an informatics department or working with the CNIO on specific projects?

■ Once you have made this decision, start your job search.

- Other than searching websites, what other activities do you need to complete? Do you have a network?

- Decide who and what you would do in the job interview and make a list.

- Review readings from the research previously discussed to gain a better understating of industry skill and competency requirements.

SUMMARY

The purpose of this chapter was to provide some of the nursing roles the APRN can assume today, if he or she has the skills needed to meet expectations identified in the job descriptions. It also provided an overview, including a partial list of role expectations needed as a PM. The following chapters provide the knowledge, tools, and recommendations on how to acquire and develop the skills needed to assume the role of PM or apply a framework needed to complete a practicum in graduate school courses. It will provide opportunities to practice using the tools, methodology, and processes inherent in each phase of the project—from designing, planning, implementing, monitoring, and controlling the project and, finally, closing the project and conducting an evaluation of the process or lessons learned. Today's workforce is expected to possess higher level knowledge and skills in order to be competent and competitive in the job market.

REFERENCES

Abu Raddaha, A. (2017). *Nurses' characteristics and perceptions toward using the electronic health record system as predictors of clinical nursing performance improvement. Clinical Nursing Studies, 5*(4), 32–41. doi:10.5430/cns.v5n4p32

American Association of Colleges of Nursing. (2011). *The essentials of master's education in nursing.* Retrieved from https://www.aacnnursing.org/Portals/42/Publications/MastersEssentials11.pdf

American Association of Colleges of Nursing. (2018). *AACN Essentials Updates.* Retrieved from https://www.aacnnursing.org/Education-Resources/AACN-Essentials

American Nurses Association. (2008). *Nursing informatics: Scope and standards of practice.* Silver Spring, MD: Nursesbooks.org.

American Nurses Association. (2015). *Nursing informatics: Scope and standards of practice* (2nd ed.). Silver Spring, MD: Nursesbooks.org.

American Nurses Association. (2016). *Nursing administration: Scope and standards of practice* (2nd ed.). Silver Spring, MD: Nursesbooks.org.

American Nurses Credentialing Center. (n.d.). Retrieved from http://www.nursecredential ing.org

American Organization of Nurse Executives. (2015). *AONE nurse executive competencies*. Chicago, IL: Author. Retrieved from https://www.aonl.org/sites/default/files/ aone/nurse-executive-competencies.pdf

American Recovery and Reinvestment Act Initiative. (2014). *HITECH act*. Retrieved from http://www.healthit.gov/policy-researchers-implementers/hitech-act

Association of College and Research Libraries. (2014). *Advancing learning, transforming scholarship: What is computer literacy?* Retrieved from http://www.ala. org/acrl/issues

Barrow, J. M., & Toney-Butler, T. J. (2019). *Change management*. Treasure Island, FL: StatPearls Publishing. Retrieved from https://www.ncbi.nlm.nih.gov/books/NBK459380

Benner, P. (1982). From novice to expert. *American Journal of Nursing, 82*(3), 402–407. Retrieved from https://journals.lww.com/ajnonline/Citation/1982/82030/From_ Novice_To_Expert.4.aspx

Benner, P. (2004). Using the Dreyfus model of skill acquisition to describe and interpret skill acquisition and clinical judgment in nursing practice and education. *Bulletin of Science, Technology and Society, 24*(3), 188–199. doi:10.1177/0270467

von Bertalanffy, L. (1968). *General system theory: Foundations, development, applications*. New York, NY: George Braziller.

Blum, B. L. (Ed.). (1986). *Clinical information systems*. New York, NY: Springer.

Bush, G. W. (2004, January 20). *State of the union address*. Retrieved from https:// georgewbush-whitehouse.archives.gov/news/releases/2004/01/20040120-7.html

Chinn, P., & Kramer, M. (2011). *Integrated theory and knowledge development in nursing* (8th ed.). St. Louis: Elsevier Mosby.

Clinical Informatics RSS Feed. (2014). *2017 Nursing Informatics Workforce Survey | HIMSS*. Retrieved from https://www.himss.org/ni-workforce-survey

Clinical Nurse Specialist: Job Description, Duties and Requirements. (2018). Retrieved from https://study.com/articles/Clinical_Nurse_Specialist_Job_Description_Duties _and_Requirements.html

Current Nursing. (2012). *Systems theory in nursing*. Retrieved from http://currentnursing. com/nursing_theory/systems_theory_in_nursing.html

Dreyfus, S., & Dreyfus, H. (1980). *A five-stage model of the mental activities involved in directed skill acquisition*. Berkeley: California University Berkeley Operations Research Center.

Foster, M., & Sethares, K. (2017, Fall). Current strategies to implement informatics into the nursing curriculum: An integrative review. *Online Journal of Nursing Informatics, 21*(3). Retrieved from https://www.himss.org/library/current-strategies-implement -informatics-nursing-curriculum-integrative-review

Fulton, C. R., Meek, J. A., & Walker, P. H. (2014). Faculty and organizational characteristics associated with informatics/health information technology adoption in DNP programs. *Journal of Professional Nursing, 30*(4), 292–299. doi:10.1016/j.profnurs .2014.01.004

Gardner, C., & Jones, S. (2012, June). Utilization of academic electronic medical records in undergraduate nursing education. *Online Journal of Nursing Informatics, 16*(2). Retrieved from http://ojni.org/issues/?p=1702

Healthcare Information and Management Systems Society. (2014). *Chief nursing information officer (CNIO) job descriptions*. Retrieved from https://www.himss.org/ sites/himssorg/files/himss-cnio-job-description.pd

Healthcare Information and Management Systems Society. (2017). *2017 nursing informatics workforce survey*. Retrieved from https://www.himss.org/ni-workforce-survey

Healthcare Information and Management Systems Society. (2018). Nursing Informatics 101. Retrieved from https://www.himss.org/file/1277691/download?token=s5UJ4dkX.

Institute of Medicine. (2011). *The future of nursing: Leading change, advancing health, better data collection and improved information infrastructure.* Washington, DC: National Academies Press.

Institute of Medicine. (2012). *Health IT and patient safety: Building safer systems for better care.* Washington, DC: National Academies Press.

Kaminski, J. (2011, Winter). Theory applied to informatics—Lewin's Change Theory. *Canadian Journal of Nursing Informatics, 6*(1). Retrieved from http://cjni.net/journal/?p=1210

Matney, S., Avant, K., & Staggers, N. (2015). Toward an understanding of wisdom in nursing. *The Online Journal of Issues in Nursing, 21*(1), 7. doi:10.3912/OJIN.Vol21No01PPT02

Matney, S., Brewster, P., Sward, K., Cloyes, K., & Staggers, N. (2011). Philosophical approaches to the nursing informatics data–information–knowledge–wisdom framework. *Advances in Nursing Science, 34*(1), 6–18. doi:10.1097/ANS.0b013e3182071813

Medscape. (2014). *Role of the advanced practice nurse.* Retrieved from https://www.medscape.com

Mohammadi, M. M., Poursaberi, R., & Salahshoor, M. R. (2018). Evaluating the adoption of evidence-based practice using Rogers's diffusion of innovation theory: A model testing study. *Health Promotion Perspectives, 8*(1), 25–32. doi:10.15171/hpp.2018.03

National Council of State Boards of Nursing (n.d.). APRNs in the U.S. Retrieved from https://www.ncsbn.org/aprn.htm

NI Toolbox and NI Knowledge Repository. (2014). Retrieved from http://www.himss.org/ni

Nilsen, P. (2015). Making sense of implementation theories, models and frameworks. *Implementation Science, 10*, 53. doi:10.1186/s13012-015-0242-0

Office of the National Coordinator for Health Information Technology. (2014). *Implementation of EHRs: Meaningful use.* Retrieved from http://dashboard.healthit.gov/quickstats/pages/FIG-MU-Hospitals-Public-Health-Measure-Attestations.htm

Project Management Institute. (2013). *A guide to the project management body of knowledge (PMBOK® Guide),* (5th ed., p. 5). Newtown Square, PA: Author.

Provost, L. (2018). *Quality improvement in healthcare: 5 guiding principles.* Retrieved from https://www.healthcatalyst.com/insights/quality-improvement-healthcare-5-guiding-principles

Reed, P. G., & Shearer, N. B. C. (2013). *Perspectives on nursing theory.* Philadelphia: Wolters Kluwer.

Research Gate. (2014). *Is project management essential for charge nurses, head nurses, nursing supervisors, and in other managerial nursing positions?* Retrieved from https://www.researchgate.net/post/Is_project_management_essential_for_charge_nurses_head_nurses_nursing_supervisors_and_in_other_managerial_nursing_positions

Risjord, M. (2009). Rethinking concept analysis. *Journal of Advanced Nursing, 65*(3), 684–691. doi:10.1111/j.1365-2648.2008.04903.x

Ronquillo, C., Currie, L. M., & Rodney, P. (2016). The evolution of data-information-knowledge-wisdom in nursing informatics. *ANS Advances in Nursing Science, 39*(1), E1–18. doi:10.1097/ANS.0000000000000107

Sipes, C. (2016). *Project management for the advance practice nurse.* New York, NY: Springer Publishing Company.

Staggers, N., & Thompson, C. B. (2002). The evolution of definitions for nursing informatics: A critical analysis and revised definition. *Journal of the American Medical Informatics Association: JAMIA, 9*(3), 255–261. doi:10.1197/jamia.M0946

U.S. Department of Health and Human Services. (2014). *What skills are needed to implement and support an EHR system?* Retrieved from http://www.hrsa.gov/healthit/toolbox/RuralHealthITtoolbox/index.html

Walker, L. O., & Avant, K. C. (2011). *Strategies for theory construction in nursing* (5th ed.). Upper Saddle River, NJ: Prentice Hall.

Zaccagnini, M., & White, K. (2017). *The doctor of nursing practice essentials: A new model for advanced practice nursing.* Sudbury, MA: Jones & Bartlett.

SECTION II

PHASES OF PROJECT MANAGEMENT

CHAPTER 3

DESIGN/INITIATION: PROJECT MANAGEMENT— PHASE 1

LEARNING OBJECTIVES

Upon completion of this chapter, the reader will be able to:

1. Discuss different types of projects.
2. Describe components of a gap analysis.
3. Define *charter*.
4. Define *scope*.
5. Describe three topics defined in a charter.
6. Describe two tasks found in a scope document.
7. Discuss three metrics and how they would be used in the project document.
8. List two items that need to be included in a measurable objective.

OUTLINE

- Key Terms
- Introduction
- Gap Analysis

- Types of Projects
- Project Goals and Objectives
- Project Charter
- Scope and Scope Creep
- Statement-of-Work Criteria
- Project Timeline
- Organizational Structures: Pros and Cons
- Stakeholders
- Team Selection and Formation
- PM Roles and Responsibilities
- Summary

KEY TERMS

- Charter
- Current state
- Design/initiation phase
- Functional organization
- Future state
- Gap analysis
- Goals
- Matrix organization
- Scope
- SMART objectives
- Stakeholder analysis
- Statement of work (SOW)
- Timeline
- Types of projects

INTRODUCTION

The role of the project manager (PM) is critical to the success of a project. Many times leadership may overlook the value of a PM, with the belief that another person in a leadership role can also assume the PM role while also completing his or her other duties. It is important to note that the role of the PM is and should be different from the operations of other functional managers. "Each functional manager is responsible for a particular division, section or project. The functional manager is usually selected for his technical expertise and ability to control the day-to-day operations of the division" (Benjamin, 2018, para. 2). As a seasoned PM, the advanced practice registered nurse (APRN) will bring skills and knowledge to the project, including a thorough understanding of the key concepts and principles of project management and leadership as well as the various skills possessed by an advanced practice clinician, which include nursing informatics skills; combining these skill sets and knowledge enables the APRN PM to facilitate and tie these together.

This chapter provides an overview of the different steps/phases in a project. The first of the five phases of a project is the design/initiation phase. The initiation process starts when it has been determined by leadership that a new project or update to an existing project is needed and the type of project is determined. The initiation phase includes conducting all the activities necessary to begin formally planning the project, which is the second step or phase. The initiation phase typically begins with the assignment of the PM, hiring of the project team, and ends when the project team has the information needed to begin developing a detailed plan and budget. At this point, the project team moves to phase 2—planning, which is discussed in Chapter 4, Planning: Project Management—Phase 2.

Activities required during the design/initiation phase include identifying the project sponsor and developing the scope and charter documents that, when signed off by leadership, formally authorize the project. This is the phase where the initial timeline for the project is developed, when the need for the project is clearly justified and defined, and measurable project objectives, including metrics, are developed.

Depending on the type of project, if part of an ongoing organizational implementation of an electronic health record (EHR) system, the initiation phase will include a review of past lessons learned to determine what went well. This is also the phase where the stakeholders need to be defined.

The stakeholders are those who have an interest in the project, such as leadership, finance, end users, project sponsors, and project team members, to name a few. At this point, it will be important to request representatives for end users, as there may be many—such as staff nurses—who may have differing ideas of what should be accomplished with the project. The stakeholders will define what the project should accomplish, such as the deliverables, which may be new clinical documentation, administrative system, pharmacy system, or an entire new system for the whole enterprise-wide organization. They will also help define the assumptions, critical success factors (CSFs), timeline, and resources. High-level stakeholders, such as a vice president, "C" levels (chief executive officer [CEO], chief informatics officer [CIO], chief nursing informatics officer [CNIO], and chief financial officer [CFO]), or other leadership, will help define the project budget and other needed aspects of the new system.

It will be important to understand the organizational philosophy for project management, whether it has a methodology, and what the PM role will be, including levels of authority and accountability. All of these tasks need to be clearly defined and then entered into project management documents during the planning phase, prior to the Kick-Off meeting that formally launches the project.

> ▶ **QUESTIONS TO CONSIDER BEFORE READING ON**
>
> 1. What is the purpose of a gap analysis?
> 2. Discuss two major steps when conducting a gap analysis.
> 3. What is a metric? How do you use metrics?
> 4. How would you develop a measurable objective?

GAP ANALYSIS

Current State

The first step when planning and launching any project is to conduct and analyze the "current state." Current state refers to reviewing the "what is"—what is currently happening—and then looking to define what and/or where the gaps might be—what is missing or what could make it better.

For example, one of the reasons a project might have been proposed is the need for a remodel, an upgrade, to solve some problem, such as long patient wait times, or to add something new that would expedite a process. Overall, the project is being implemented to meet a need, and the need or gap should be justified with documentation of workflows to show the gaps. These shapes and maps can be drawn using such programs as Microsoft Visio, PowerPoint, or OpenOffice.org Draw.

When beginning to diagram a workflow, the first step is to start by drawing boxes that will represent each step in the process until arriving at a step where there is a gap in the flow—the gap analysis (see Figure 3.1), which clearly shows the gaps in the process. It is important to do this first by just sketching the diagram quickly on a notepad while working with others who may be providing information so that thought processes are not lost. As frequently happens, the process will include a review and may be revised a number of times. As end users start to think through the processes, with repeated reviews they will begin to remember more details, especially if they are working with others to document the workflow. After several iterations have been completed, the diagram can be formally documented, especially using a program called Microsoft Visio. If one is not familiar with this program, there may be a steep learning curve to learn how to use it, but there may be no time to do so. Many times organizations have someone on the project who has experience using the application.

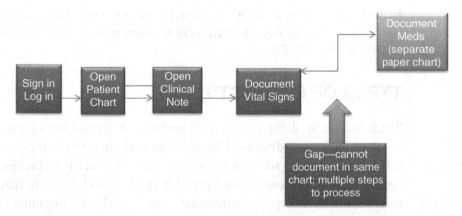

FIGURE 3.1 Current-state electronic clinical documentation with a gap in charting.
SOURCE: Sipes, C. (2016). *Project management for the advanced practice nurse.* New York, NY: Springer Publishing Company.

Documentation of the gap analysis is conducted to define what parts of the workflow process are not working well, which are taking too much time, such as redundant charting, or other steps in the process that may cause extra work. This process review may be able to identify a missing application that will greatly speed up a process or function.

Future State

The next step is to design the "future-state" application. There are many considerations when implementing the future state or "what will be," such as the impact and change the new process will cause the entire organization. Change can be very difficult; most people do not like change and are content with the status quo. Change management techniques and plan as well as tool development are discussed in Chapter 4, Planning: Project Management—Phase 2, and Chapter 5, Implementation/Execution—Phase 3. The future-state diagrams will show the new changes in the workflow and where the proposed changes will occur (see Figure 3.2).

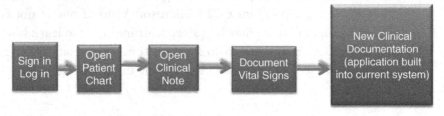

FIGURE 3.2 Future-state electronic clinical documentation: gap resolved.
SOURCE: Sipes, C. (2016). *Project management for the advanced practice nurse.* New York, NY: Springer Publishing Company.

TYPES OF PROJECTS

There are many different types of projects. A partial list of potential types of projects is discussed here. These include quality improvement (QI); optimization (additions after the initial project is implemented); applications of evidence-based practice (EBP); small projects that may include one or two application updates, such as clinical documentation; integration of "legacy" (old) to the new EHR system; and others. These all have a variety of timelines, resources, and other components that fall under the definition of a project because they are temporary, as there is an end once the project is completed. The QI types of project and EBP are further defined in Chapter 6, Monitoring and Controlling: Project Management—Phase 4. Examples of activities associated with these projects, QI and EBP, are presented.

PROJECT GOALS AND OBJECTIVES

Critical to the detail in project management documents is the inclusion of measurable, well-defined goals and objectives. A "goal" is defined as a general statement about some task or project that needs to be accomplished, such as this new EHR will "go live" in 10 months. The objectives define the specific steps that determine how the goal(s) will be accomplished, how to get there and help keep the project moving. To do this a number of key tracking tools need to be developed and questions answered as in the following list. Many PMs who create management documents find it difficult to develop well-defined, specific goals and objectives, only to discover later that they were missing a task, due date, or owner of a specific task and therefore cannot adequately track whether this missing item has been completed. One thing to remember is that the project management tools developed need to be tracked many times every week and updated to meet the evolution of the project as it begins to take shape.

Even the official scope document can be amended if well justified that some critical element was overlooked and agreed to by all of leadership and stakeholders. Key to better understanding of tracking critical elements is to assure they are measurable using well-defined metrics. Well-defined metrics include the use of numbers (how many of XXX)—percentages; due dates; comparisons; budgets; number of staff, patients, and departments; units of measure; and many others—that can be tracked, analyzed, and modified (Business Dictionary, 2018).

- Number of units: How many applications will be included in the new system?
- Specific tasks to be completed: Design of system (who does this?), build (how long?), and testing (which ones?).
- Due dates: Due date for phase 1 completion, phases 2, 3, 4, and 5? Go-live date?
- Owners/responsibility: Who are the stakeholders? Who builds the system? And so on. Each task will be assigned a responsible owner to make sure it is completed and passes all tests.

Each of the preceding items will need a metric—a number—so that percentage of completion can be tracked and measured each week. You can think of a well-defined objective by answering the five W questions of who, what, where, when, and why and an H question of how (Sipes, 2016).

- Who and what department or role needs to do the activities?
- Who will the project impact?
- Who will pay for the project?
- Who is making the decisions?
- What are the benefits, and to whom?
- Where will this occur—regional, enterprise wide, or one specific hospital?
- When will the different activities be completed?
- Why is this project being done?
- How will this be completed—list of tasks, resources? (Sipes, 2016)

Writing SMART Objectives

The objectives should be developed as SMART objectives, meaning they need to be *specific, measurable, achievable (attainable), relevant, and timely* (Table 3.1; Landau, 2018).

The key to developing critical measurable objectives is having collectable data that are adequate for measuring change (Issel & Wells, 2018).

TABLE 3.1 Goal and SMART Objectives

GOAL	IMPLEMENT STAFF TRAINING PROJECT FOR NURSING DEPARTMENT
▪ S = Specific; answer the five W questions	▪ The training for the clinical documentation application in the EHR will be implemented for the 5N Medical–Surgical Nursing department. ▪ Training will start on March 15, 2019, by staff super-user trainers prior to the system going live.
▪ M = Measurable; how will you know when you have accomplished the objective?	▪ The education will be accomplished when 35 RN staff from 5N the Medical–Surgical Nursing department complete and pass the training. ▪ They will need to pass the competency test with 85% within 2 weeks of completing the training that starts on March 15, 2019, and ends on March 30, 2019.

(continued)

TABLE 3.1 Goal and SMART Objectives (*continued*)

GOAL	IMPLEMENT STAFF TRAINING PROJECT FOR NURSING DEPARTMENT
■ A = Achievable; will you be able to achieve it within the multiple constraints—time, budget, resources, quality, and risk?	■ The time allotted to complete the training was approved by leadership on February 1. ■ The budget to complete the training was approved by leadership on February 1. ■ Three additional trainers have been hired and completed their training on March 1.
■ R = Relevant; do the objectives comply with the organization's mission?	■ The objectives comply with the organization's mission goals of implementing an EHR in NM Health Systems in 2019, to improve patient safety and access to healthcare.
■ T = Timely; do you have due dates for every task?	■ Metrics for each objective are included, for example, the number of staff, number of trainers, location, and due dates.

EHR, electronic health record; RN, registered nurse.

SOURCES: Sipes, C. (2016). *Project management for the advanced practice nurse.* New York, NY: Springer Publishing Company. Adapted from cdc.gov. (2009). *Writing SMART objectives.* Retrieved from https://www.cdc.gov/healthyyouth/evaluation/pdf/brief3b.pdf; Landau, P. (2018). How to create SMART goals. *ProjectManagement.com.* Retrieved from https://www.projectmanager.com/blog/how-to-create-smart-goals

CASE SCENARIO 3.1

Laura is completing her graduate project in project management and nursing informatics. Her assignment is to prepare a scope document that has goals and measureable objectives. She starts to discuss the assignment with other classmates and realizes she does not understand what a metric is and asks, "Where is the formula we are supposed to use?"

She starts to complete a literature search to find examples on how to use metrics but can find no "formulas."

■ How would you explain what metrics are and how to use them?

■ How would using the SMART process help Laura?

> ▶ **QUESTIONS TO CONSIDER BEFORE READING ON**
> 1. What is the purpose of a project charter?
> 2. How is a project charter different from the scope document?
> 3. What is scope creep?
> 4. How will you mitigate scope creep?

PROJECT CHARTER

What Is a Charter?

In this phase of design, a number of key project management documents are created, including the charter, which adds the framework for the who, what, when, why, where, and how, so the project can proceed, including the formal sign-off by key leadership and stakeholders, which authorizes the project and gives authority to the PM. A needs assessment, also referred to as the "workflow gap analysis," includes a review of the current state of the project as well as anticipated future-state information. The workflow analysis helps to define and organize basic draft ideas into a more comprehensive format that is easier to follow. The needs assessment contains the evaluation of the business need for the project as well as the anticipated outcome of the project. According to Ray (2017), the project charter is "the statement of scope, objectives and people who are participating in a project. It begins the process of defining the roles and responsibilities of those participants and outlines the objectives and goals of the project. The charter also identifies the main stakeholders and defines the authority of the project manager" (para. 1).

The project charter is based on the outcomes of the gap analysis; it also defines costs, lists tasks in the form of a schedule, and contains a Gantt chart and the deliverables. The charter is different from the scope document. The project charter has one primary purpose: to authorize a PM to use defined resources to complete a project and assign a project sponsor. The scope document is prepared (along with the charter and other initiation documents) to map out the goals. A well-written scope statement clearly defines the boundaries of a project (Maciver, 2018, p. 1).

To develop a project charter, you will need to identify the information found in Table 3.2.

TABLE 3.2 Project Charter Content

PROJECT CHARTER		
Title of project:		
Objective of project:		
Background/justification:		
Scope statement summary:		
Project participants:		
Executive Steering Team (EST)		
Name	Title	Department
Roles and responsibilities:		
Time requirement:		
Total estimated hours per member:		
Project Steering Team (PST)		
Name	Title	Department
Roles and responsibilities:		
Time requirement:		
Total estimated hours per member:		
Project Work Team		
Name	Title	Department
Project governance:		
Roles and responsibilities:		
Time requirement:		
Total estimated hours per member:		
Other resources: (vendors; administrative, clinical, technical resources that will be required)		
Activities: (will be listed in project plan)		
Deliverables: (to support scope document)		
Time frame:		
Special considerations: (assumptions, constraints, directives from management)		
Approval and sign-off: (project sponsor agrees with scope of activities and deliverables)		
Name	Title	Department

SOURCE: Sipes, C. (2016). *Project management for the advanced practice nurse.* New York, NY: Springer Publishing Company.

SCOPE AND SCOPE CREEP

The scope document is a formal document that details how the project will be managed and what the project requirements are. It defines the boundaries of what can and cannot be done. After the scope document is approved by key stakeholders, any additional or further change will need to go through the change management process (described in Chapter 4, Planning: Project Management—Phase 2, and Chapter 5, Implementation/Execution—Phase 3) and be approved again by stakeholders and other key leadership. The scope document should address the problem or opportunity that will be resolved with the implementation of the project. It defines the project goal and objectives and the metrics that will be used to determine the success of the project (Team Clarizen, 2017, 2018). When the scope document is completed, it will need to be included as one document with the charter.

Mitigating Scope Creep

Unapproved change in scope—known as "scope creep"—can cause delays in the project and/or budget overruns, especially if there are issues such as acquiring additional human and other resources, such as equipment. Scope creep occurs when something is forgotten and not included in the original requirements document but must be itemized and then added to the project scope but not always approved prior to adding. The two major components that need to be evaluated in scope creep are:

- Define the extent of the project change, such as costs, resources, and time
- Complete an assessment of the impact of the change on the organization

To determine how changes will impact the project, different attributes will need to be analyzed and documented. Those include, but are not limited to:

- The type of impact the change will have
- Impact on project schedule and timeline
- Whether the project can incorporate and accommodate the change
- What will happen to the project if the change is not implemented
- How manageable the change is—time, cost, resources, quality

The CSFs will also need to be defined, including a timeline for completion of all deliverables. Content that will need to be included in the scope statement is listed in Table 3.3.

TABLE 3.3 Scope Statement

Organization's name:		
Project's name:		
Scope document:		
Project manager:	Priority level: Low, Medium, High	
Sponsors:		
Mission statement:		
Measurable project objectives:		
Justification:		
Implementation strategy:		
Project resources:		
Completion date:		
Measures of success/critical success factors:		
Assumptions:		
Constraints:		
	Stakeholder/Leadership Approvals	
Manager and sponsor:	Signatures:	Date:
Project manager approval:		
Owner approval:		

SOURCE: Sipes, C. (2016). *Project management for the advanced practice nurse.* New York, NY: Springer Publishing Company.

Difference Between a Charter and Scope: Getting Approval

A project charter defines the purpose of the project and includes measurable objectives (see Table 3.1). It also includes a list of the high-level requirements for the project as well as the project description. It should include expected milestones and a budget. It includes the PM's job description, with definitions of the roles and responsibilities, and clearly defines the authority levels, including reporting structure. Finally, it lists who the authorizing person(s) is and includes requirements for how different aspects of the project will be approved.

In contrast, the scope document includes a description of the project and defines the project deliverables (a product or service). It defines what is in scope and what is not included in the scope of the project. It also defines the user acceptance criteria and includes constraints and assumptions for the project (Table 3.4).

TABLE 3.4 Key Differences Between a Charter and Scope Statement

PROJECT SCOPE	PROJECT CHARTER
■ Describes project	■ Includes the purpose and description of the project
■ Specifies project deliverables	■ Outlines measurable objectives and expected milestones
■ Specifies what is in scope and what is not included	■ Defines high-level requirements
■ Defines the user acceptance criteria	■ Lists approval requirements; sign-off authorizes the project
■ Lists constraints	■ Defines the project manager's roles and responsibilities and the reporting structure
■ Lists assumptions	■ Contains the budget

SOURCE: Adapted from Project Charter vs. Scope Statement. June 6, 2014 by Bernie Roseke, https://www.projectengineer.net/project-charter-vs-scope-statement

CASE SCENARIO 3.2

Susan, a nurse manager on the cardiac ICU unit, has been assigned to be the project manager (PM) for a new EHR system the organization she works for has just approved. She has some management experience, but she is not sure she understands all that is needed as a PM. She asks the director for some suggestions.

The director refers her to the newly hired CNIO who has project management experience from previous implementation where she was involved. The CNIO states she will support Susan in her new role but she also needs to work with a consultant who has many years of expertise managing new EHR implementations.

The consultant has given Susan a list of "tools" she needs to develop for the different phases of the project.

Starting with Phase 1:

■ Scope and charter

■ Statement of work (SOW)

■ Tasks with metrics

(continued)

- Due/end dates (timelines) for all phases of the project
- Implementation dates

Susan is not sure what all these documents entail so she starts to develop draft documents of these while consulting both the consultant and the CNIO.

STATEMENT-OF-WORK CRITERIA

If the organization or project requires an SOW, it can be one of the most important things that you might need to develop in place of the project charter and scope documents. However, many of the other documents you will develop as a PM would be redundant if you are also required to create and include an SOW. This informational note is only included here as some organizations do require all documents, especially government organizations. An SOW will include:

- Background, requirements, and history of proposed project
- Charter documents
- Scope document
- Objectives of the project
- Tasks to be completed in the project
- Project schedule
- Project milestones
- Deliverables of the project
- Resource management and budget

The SOW will include the documented five Ws and an H—who, what, where, why, when, and how (Sipes, 2016). The SOW is a legal contract between a number of contractors, the organization, and leadership. Some organizations require that you also include the assumptions found in the scope. When this document is completed, it will need to be reviewed by legal advisors and leadership for approval and sign-off as approval for the project to proceed.

PROJECT TIMELINE

The project timeline is another extremely important document that must be developed at the outset of a project. This document provides a quick view of the overall project and includes high-level milestones to be completed each week or month, depending on the length of the project. This document should be reviewed at every weekly project and stakeholder meeting to validate the project is on track.

Many organizations keep a large wall map of a timeline, such as the timeline shown in Figure 3.3, as a constant reminder of where the project is and where it is going. Frequently, the timeline includes detail to keep team members and others who are involved in the project informed; it is a key to good communication.

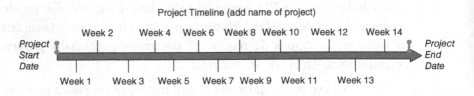

FIGURE 3.3 Project timeline.
SOURCE: Sipes, C. (2016). *Project management for the advanced practice nurse.* New York, NY: Springer Publishing Company.

ORGANIZATIONAL STRUCTURES: PROS AND CONS

Functional Organizations

Functional organizations are the most common organizations you might see or be involved with. These organizations are organized more by function, such as an information technology (IT) department. A disadvantage of this type of organization is that communication tends to flow from the top down through the organization—from CEO down through the vice presidents (VPs) to the managers, and then staff.

A typical functional organization chart might look like the example shown in Figure 3.4.

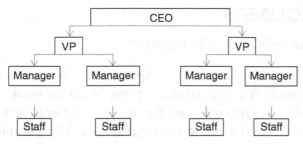

FIGURE 3.4 Functional organization.
SOURCE: Sipes, C. (2014). *Developing measureable objectives: Using the five Ws (document in NR 640, 642 and 643)*. Downers Grove, IL: Chamberlain College of Nursing.

Matrix Organizations

A matrix organization takes advantage of staff who might be working on several projects at a time, and therefore would be reporting to both the functional managers and the PMs for their projects.

Within a matrix organization, the power is shared between the two PMs as shown in Figure 3.5.

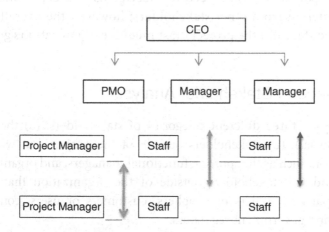

FIGURE 3.5 Matrix organization.
PMO, project management office.
SOURCE: Sipes, C. (2014). *Developing measureable objectives: Using the five Ws (document in NR 640, 642 and 643)*. Downers Grove, IL: Chamberlain College of Nursing.

Can you see any potential problems with having to share resources across several different projects?

STAKEHOLDERS

Project Stakeholder Management

It will be very important to keep key stakeholders involved in the project informed, as a key stakeholder can "make or break" a project. A "stakeholder" is someone who has a vested interest in the project or can be the greatest critic in the organization. The PM must engage stakeholders, manage expectations, and ensure that the project gets what it needs from stakeholders, and stakeholders get what they need from the project. As the stakeholders are identified, it is important that significant requirements are captured, documented, and incorporated in order to engage stakeholders and manage their expectations. The sooner they are identified, the better the opportunity to gain support and mitigate risks—timely and frequent communication is crucial. More on managing stakeholder expectations, including addressing their needs, communication, and status meetings, is covered in Chapter 5, Implementation/Execution—Phase 3.

Each stakeholder for the project may have different goals. For each of their departments, they need to meet goals and expectations that will be different from other stakeholders; however, the overall goal of the stakeholders and the project must meet the organization's goals and mission.

Importance of Stakeholder Analysis

There may be three different categories of stakeholders: (a) the project team (internal); (b) stakeholders outside of the project, but within the organization, such as the sponsor, functional managers, and organizational groups; and (c) stakeholders outside of the organization that include business partners, sellers or suppliers, customers or users, community interests, and government regulators.

It will be important to develop a matrix to define which stakeholders "own" certain parts of the project—include the project team members as this is developed. If important stakeholders are not included in the project, they may not support the project when it is needed or may even interfere with the project, potentially leading to project failure. Stakeholders' goals may be affected by the project, either positively or negatively, even though they are not actually involved in the project. For all of these reasons, it will be crucial to have a documented process for elevating *any* change—that there is a change control board (CCB) and that all changes go through the review and approval process.

The team will develop a matrix starting with one side that will reflect those who support the project. There are many examples of matrices and how to use them to your advantage available on the web, YouTube, and others, but a simple example is shown in Figure 3.6.

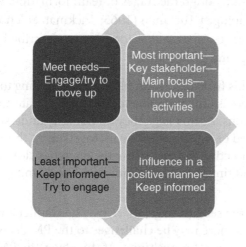

FIGURE 3.6 Stakeholder analysis.
SOURCE: Sipes, C. (2016). *Project management for the advanced practice nurse.* New York, NY: Springer Publishing Company.

TEAM SELECTION AND FORMATION

The team members selected for the project will depend on the type of organization and the need for specific applications, such as clinical documentation and medication order entry. Team members for these applications include nurses, physicians, and pharmacists. As the teams are formed, necessary skills of potential team members are evaluated. If nurses are needed but the nurses lack analytical skills, they may be sent to the vendor for training. If this type of training—as an analyst—is required, this will need to be added into the project budget. According to Satell's (2018) *4 Ways to Build an Innovative Team*, one of the most important keys to success was that what mattered most to team performance was "psychological safety, or the ability of each team member to be able to give voice to their ideas without fear of reprisal or rebuke" (para. 9).

Organizing teams can be a challenge. Much depends on whether potential members have worked together in the past and, if so, how successful the collaboration was. It would be a big advantage for the APRN if a group of nurses worked together on the same unit and now will work together on a clinical implementation. As other members are added to the team, there may be more movement through the stages of team formation, which was first described by psychologist Tuckman (1965; Tuckman & Jensen, 1977). The four well-known stages of team development he described are forming, storming, norming, and performing:

- *Forming*—In this first stage, team members are getting to know each other; there is little friction and the team is polite and will offer few opinions. At this stage they do not fully understand what work is required or how each will work together. At this point the PM must be directive and make sure the team has clear objectives. It is also a good time to evaluate individual skills and personalities.

- *Storming*—In the second stage, there may be conflict among team members; there may be challenges to the PM decisions; and members may jockey for positions. At this stage, the PM may need to clarify roles if they have not been clear in the past; at this stage authority may be challenged. The APRN PMs must remember that they are ultimately responsible for the project.

- *Norming*—In the third stage, the team starts to work better together and resolve their differences; they better understand and respect their different roles as well as those of the PM. As the team moves along and as new tasks come up, there may be periods when they move back to storming as they again clarify their roles. It will be important to facilitate further collaboration among the team members.

- *Performing*—In the fourth stage, the team, without friction, moves toward accomplishing the project goals and objectives. At this point, the APRN may more easily delegate much of the work but must always remember the ultimate responsibility for the entire project lies with the PM (Tuckman, 1965).

Project management teams have added a fifth stage called "adjourning." In this stage "the project is coming to an end and the team members are moving off into different directions. This stage looks at the team from the perspective of the well-being of the team rather than from the perspective of managing a team through the original four stages of team growth" (Project-Management.com, 2018, "Stage 5"). The concepts of five stages—including *adjourning*—are also supported by the Oxford Learning Institute where they note that "If the team has been successful, this can be one of the most difficult stages. If the team has not been successful, the sense of unfinished business can create a blockage to future individual group development" (Oxford Learning Institute, 2018, p. 2).

At this point the team leader should ensure that there is time for the team to celebrate the success of the project and document best practices, or if not, what would need to be improved for future projects. Adjourning provides the team opportunities to say good-bye and good luck to each other as they pursue their next endeavor (Project Management, 2018, "Stage 5").

An important criterion when leading teams is to establish ground rules at the very start of a project; this will improve team collaboration. Schwarz (2017), an organizational psychologist, suggests that there are eight key rules that effective teams should follow in order to improve team collaboration. The eight ground rules are:

1. State views and ask genuine questions.
2. Share all relevant information.
3. Use specific examples and agree on what important words mean.
4. Explain reasoning and intent.
5. Focus on interests, not positions.
6. Test assumptions and inferences.
7. Jointly design next steps.
8. Discuss undiscussable issues (Schwarz, 2017).

The APRN as PM should then provide examples and how to use each of these rules. For example, be explicit—say "Put your cell phones on vibrate," "Step out of the room if you must take a call," "Start on time, end on time," "There is no wrong answer," "Treat each other with respect," and "Whatever you think" is not an acceptable response. There should be active engagement so that all feel as if they are contributing. These are a few of the universal ground rules seen today.

Another researcher, Pentland (2015), looked at data related to team performance and found "with remarkable consistency, the data showed that the most important predictor of a team's success was its communication patterns. Those patterns were as significant as all other factors—intelligence, personality, talent—combined." He identified three communication factors that consistently affect performance: exploration, energy, and engagement. When team members evaluated their own communication styles, they found they could dramatically improve their performance.

The APRN as PM will invariably find herself or himself in situations of conflict in spite of establishing ground rules. Managing team conflicts is a skill set the APRN will need to develop if she or he is not already experienced in resolving conflict. Most of the conflicts will be resolved easily and professionally; it is important to remember that not all conflict is bad. Understanding how to manage conflict will go a long way to dealing with it and must be done to keep the project moving forward.

First, it will be important to determine what caused the conflict, such as prioritizing a task, who should own the task, or trouble with timelines. Once the PM better understands the issues, the next step is to get the parties who are having the conflict together. There are several approaches that may lead to conflict resolution: collaboration, compromise, smoothing, withdrawing, as well as others. Each approach has pros and cons, but the key thing to remember is that the project must keep moving on (Harrian, 2018; Shonk, 2018a, 2018b; Stanleigh, 2018). Another process for managing teams is called "resource leveling," which is discussed in Chapter 4, Planning: Project Management—Phase 2.

REFLECTION QUESTIONS

The team is starting to come together, the project scope and charter documents are completed with sign-off approval, and the statement of work is competed in draft form. The team has a list of the stakeholders and is working to define who has more interest in supporting the project to see it through to completion.

A very high-level official of the state government wants to be included as a stakeholder on the project and has input but does not support the full project.

1. As a PM, what is your first responsibility? (This is a functional organization shown in Figure 3.4.)
2. Whom do you report to first?

PM ROLES AND RESPONSIBILITIES

As a PM, the APRN will need the skills required to assume the role of PM. Although the APRN may not assume a formal PM role, he or she would still apply the project management principles in his or her advanced role as a nurse manager, administrator, quality assurance manager, nursing informaticist, or student in master's and doctoral levels as he or she moves to achieve higher levels of education.

In addition to the skill sets that a PM must have, as discussed earlier, a partial list of classic functions and skills that a PM will be required to have included are the ability to:

- Manage teams responsible for delivering the project "outputs" to meet the triple constraints—on time, on budget, and in scope
- Plan, organize, monitor, and control the project as a manager
- Handle key responsibilities for developing the project plan and tracking and managing the project, including managing and directing the resources to meet the project objectives; these key responsibilities continue throughout the entire project life cycle
- Continually monitor communications to ensure clear communication with the project team and stakeholders
- Organize the project into small workable steps and monitor closely to ensure all steps are completed to meet project goals
- Design and prepare all project documents, especially scope and charter; obtain all necessary approvals and sign-offs for project deliverables
- Manage stakeholder relationships, including all end user communication and expectations for project tasks
- Work in collaboration with leadership to manage change expectations and behaviors

The project management functions that the APRN will be expected to assume are discussed in the next chapters—planning, implementation, monitor and control, and finally closing the project, conducting the final evaluation and lessons learned. Examples of the tools that the APRN will need to develop as well as the activities and examples of how to utilize them are included.

CRITICAL THINKING QUESTIONS AND ACTIVITIES

You are organizing your team and have selected five new members who have varying degrees of expertise for the different stages of the project that will be designed and implemented. They have been working together now for 1 week but you are beginning to see disagreements with some of the decision making.

1. What stage of team development is this?
2. What are some specific things you will do to help move the team forward? Where would you find this information online?
3. At what point will you know the team is moving to the next step in team formation?
4. What specifically will you do to facilitate and support the team to function better? List some activities you would use in team meetings.

SUMMARY

This chapter provides the definitions of the terms that PMs will encounter as they begin to design the project. It provides examples, tables, and figures representative of what is commonly seen in the industry and parallels the expectations of a healthcare organization, such as the current- and future-state workflow diagrams that are created first to determine where gaps in efficiency can be found. It provides examples of a scope document and a charter, which are critical documents that set the boundaries for the project. The SOW description is included because some organizations may require it in addition to the scope and charter documents. Also included is an example of a project timeline that many organizations post for all teams to see. An overview of the organizational structures is provided, as teams and PMs need to understand the hierarchy and management philosophy of the organization.

Finally, team selection and formation criteria are provided, along with typical team behaviors that the APRN PM needs to understand in order to have a well-functioning team. The four phases of team behaviors are forming, storming, norming, and performing. There are also suggestions for managing team conflicts and the methods to use to resolve them. Examples of PM roles and responsibilities that may be encountered in a variety of healthcare settings are also provided. Although PM roles may vary by setting, the project management concepts and principles will always apply. Many explanations and tools provided in this chapter support and help the APRN, who is beginning to assume the PM role.

REFERENCES

Benjamin, T. (2018). *What is the difference between a strategic manager & a functional manager?* Retrieved from http://smallbusiness.chron.com/difference-between -strategic-manager-functional-manager-35884.html

Business Dictionary. (2018). What are metrics? Definition and meaning. *BusinessDictionary.com.* Retrieved from http://www.businessdictionary.com/ definition/metrics.html

Harrian, E. (2018). *How to resolve conflict on projects.* Retrieved from https://www .thebalancecareers.com/how-to-resolve-project-conflicts-4105016

Issel, M., & Wells, R. (2018). *Health program planning and evaluation: A practical, systematic approach for community health* (4th ed., pp. 11–13). Boston, MA: Jones & Bartlett.

Landau, P. (2018). *How to create SMART goals* [Blog post]. Retrieved from https://www .projectmanager.com/blog/how-to-create-smart-goals

Maciver, D. (2018). *The difference between project charter and project scope statement* [Blog post]. Retrieved from https://www.barvas.com/resources/blog/the-difference -between-project-charter-and-project-scope-statement

Oxford Learning Institute. (2018). *Stages in group development; one model.* Retrieved from https://www.learning.ox.ac.uk/media/global/wwwadminoxacuk/localsites/oxford learninginstitute/documents/supportresources/lecturersteachingstaff/development programmes/StagesinGroupDevelopment.pdf

Pentland, A. (2015). The new science of building great teams. *Harvard Business Review,* 60–70. Retrieved from https://emergentcognition.com/2015/03/27/alex-sandy -pentland-harvard-business-review-the-new-science-of-building-great-teams

Project-Management.com. (2018). The five stages of project team development. Retrieved from https://www.project-management.com/the-five-stages-of-project -team-development

Ray, S. (2017). *A quick guide to project charters* [Blog post]. Retrieved from https:// www.projectmanager.com/blog/project-charter

Satell, G. (2018). 4 ways to build an innovative team. *Harvard Business Review.* Retrieved from https://hbr.org/2018/02/4-ways-to-build-an-innovative-team

Schwarz, R. (2017). *The skilled facilitator: A comprehensive resource for consultants, facilitators, managers, trainers, and coaches* (3rd ed., pp. 3–12). San Francisco, CA: Jossey-Bass.

Shonk, K. (2018a). *Conflict resolution: 3 types of conflict and how to address them* [Blog post]. Retrieved from https://www.pon.harvard.edu/daily/conflict-resolution/types -conflict

Shonk, K. (2018b). *Conflict resolution: Dealing with difficult people? Negotiation lessons from Ronald Reagan* [Blog post]. Retrieved from https://www.pon.harvard.edu/daily/ conflict-resolution/dealing-with-difficult-people-lessons-from-ronald-reagan

Sipes, C. (2014). *Developing measureable objectives: Using the five Ws (document in NR 640, 642 and 643).* Downers Grove, IL: Chamberlain College of Nursing.

Sipes, C. (2016). *Project management for the advanced practice nurse.* New York, NY: Springer Publishing Company.

Stanleigh, M. (2018). *Dealing with conflict in project teams*. Retrieved from https://bia
.ca/dealing-with-conflict-in-project-teams-2

Team Clarizen. (2017). *Why project scope is so important* [Blog post]. Retrieved from
https://www.clarizen.com/project-scope-important

Team Clarizen. (2018). *Goal versus objective: What's the difference?* [Blog post].
Retrieved from https://www.clarizen.com/goal-vs-objective-difference

Tuckman, B. W. (1965). Developmental sequence in small groups. *Psychological
Bulletin, 63*(6), 384–399. doi:10.1037/h0022100

Tuckman, B. W., & Jensen, M. A. (1977). Stages in small group development revisited.
Group and Organisation Studies, 2, 419–427. doi:10.1177/105960117700200404

CHAPTER 4

PLANNING: PROJECT MANAGEMENT—PHASE 2

LEARNING OBJECTIVES

Upon completion of this chapter, the reader will be able to:

1. Define the steps in the planning phase.
2. Discuss three tasks to be accomplished during the planning phase.
3. Discuss the value of a work breakdown structure (WBS).
4. Explain why a responsibility/accountability matrix is needed.
5. Discuss what content should be documented in the risk plan and why.
6. Define what constraints are. Why do they need to be monitored?
7. Discuss why it is important to define and monitor critical success factors (CSFs).
8. Discuss the value of a network diagram.
9. Explain the final step in the planning phase and why it is important.

OUTLINE

- Key Terms
- Introduction
- Planning Processes
- Tools
- Project Management Skills and Competencies

- The Project Plan
- Tracking Schedules
- Building the Budget and Managing the Resources
- Project Responsibility and Accountability
- Risk Assessment and Management Plan
- Communication
- Change Management
- Deliverables and CSFs
- Importance of Status Meetings
- Kick-Off Meeting
- Summary

KEY TERMS

- Actual cost of work performed (ACWP)
- Budgeted cost of work performed (BCWP)
- Budgeted cost of work scheduled (BCWS)
- Change management
- Constraints
- Cost variance (CV)
- Critical path (CP)
- Critical success factor (CSF)
- Deliverables
- Earned value (EV)
- Fast Track
- Gantt chart
- Kick-Off meeting
- Network diagram
- Responsible, accountable, consulted, informed (RACI)
- Risk
- Schedule variance (SV)

- Statement of work (SOW)
- Status meetings
- Work breakdown structure (WBS)

INTRODUCTION

Planning Processes, Tools, and Skills Needed for the Project

After the design/initiation phase of project management comes the second, or planning, phase of a project. If the project has been approved and the key stakeholders have signed off on it, it means there is support for the planning and implementation of the project. This phase is one of the most important phases of the project. If tasks or activities are not identified and planned during this phase, it can cause delays in the overall project. If the advanced practice nurse project manager (APRN PM) does not develop the plan with great detail, it may be one of the reasons for project delay, even failure, especially if a key task was forgotten. Many times senior leadership is anxious to move quickly to implement a project by cutting the planning phase short, which may create a potential gap in the planning process and omit key deliverables needed for project success. The detailed, very specific project plan is key to setting the expectations using the five Ws and an H (Sipes, 2016): who, what, where, why, when, and how, which are needed to successfully complete the project. All of these specific details were outlined in the project objectives during the design phase and now can be revised and updated as more information regarding the project is gathered. In this chapter, the planning processes are presented as well as the tools that will need to be developed to monitor and track the project. Key to the overall success of all the activities required to implement a project are the knowledge and leadership skills needed by the PM in order to be successful.

> ▶ **QUESTIONS TO CONSIDER BEFORE READING ON**
> 1. What is the benefit of project planning?
> 2. What types of tasks are included in project planning?
> 3. What are some of the key "tools" developed during this phase?
> 4. Discuss leadership skills required to lead a project.
> 5. Discuss barriers to successful project outcomes.

PLANNING PROCESSES
Eight Steps in Project Planning

The planning steps of project management provide a road map that specifies the details necessary for the PM to support the project team so that it thrives, while the PM helps the team navigate the project highway to implement a successful project. Many of the project tasks or items build upon one another in that one may need to be completed before the next one starts. Since these are not set in stone, they can be updated to meet the identified project requirements as more information is gathered. While tasks can be modified and changed, using the process and tools developed in this phase when the change management plan is created, they require leadership input and sign-off approval when moving through the change management board, which is discussed later in this chapter. Many of the tools and their variations can be found on the web. Most organizations define their own model of how they want a project completed and have tools unique to their organizations as well. The tools here are those developed and used on a number of projects. Frequently, it has been easier for an organization to use and modify what already exists.

The project's scope and charter were developed and approved during design/initiation, the initial or first phase in Chapter 3, Design/Initiation: Project Management—Phase 1. The planning phase builds on the processes established in the design phase and now will develop the project "tool kit," including WBS, timelines, and many other tracking and monitoring tools, using the eight steps in project planning. The steps listed here are a partial list but provide a good place to start planning. The steps include:

1. Build a project scope based upon the project charter.
2. Break down the scope into tasks/work packages.
3. Assign tasks/work packages to their owners.
4. Task/work package owners build activity lists needed to complete a larger task.
5. Activity owners estimate or calculate activity durations with start/end dates.
6. As a team, all activity owners are involved in sequencing activities.
7. Identify and document dependencies; what needs to be done first.
8. Build a schedule/timeline based on steps 1 to 7.

It is important to understand which tools should be developed first so that others may follow the same format, making each subsequent tool easier and more efficient to build. Project teams often struggle with the level of detail in the tools and documents, such as the charter, saying they cannot build it yet, because they do not know enough about the project. It is important to remember that documents and tools developed during the initial phases will evolve and be updated as more information about the project is gathered. Changes can be made with approvals from all stakeholders as new information becomes available, as long as the change management process and tracking tools are used as discussed previously.

You are learning that project planning is critical to a project's success and extremely important for the project team. To be effective and efficient, a team must have a plan. Without a plan to provide structure and direction, a project can become chaotic, inadvertently consuming resources and jeopardizing the limitations set for the project, such as budget, timelines/due dates, resources, and other factors, which are discussed later in this chapter. Have you been on a project without a plan? What was the outcome?

The amount of detail and the number of components in the plan vary depending on several factors:

- Project duration
- Project complexity
- Organization's adherence to a formal project management methodology

To reinforce what was learned in Chapter 3, Design/Initiation: Project Management—Phase 1, an emphasis is on developing measurable, SMART objectives or the "five Ws and an H" for objectives, which must be very detailed in order to provide direction for the project.

TOOLS

Support Documents

The support documents and tools to be developed during the planning phase include but are not limited to:

- A WBS document; statement of work (SOW)
- Project plan with Gantt chart, which defines owners, and start and end dates for each task

- Network diagram which outlines what needs to be done first before something else is started—think "domino effect"
- Project schedules/timelines with due dates
- Communication plan
- Risk management plan
- Resource management plan

The project charter was created and approved in Chapter 3, Design/ Initiation: Project Management—Phase 1. The other project tools are developed by the project team and approved by all of the key project stakeholders unless the organization has its own tools and documents that will be required. The approval process is very important because it officially authorizes the use of resources and provides funding for the project.

Effective project teams take this approval one step further by performing a baseline assessment. The baseline is a snapshot, a quick overview, but not comprehensive, of the project at the start. It is essentially the APRN PM's estimates of:

- What tasks are included?
- What are the resources; where will they come from? Human and software/hardware
- Start dates; end dates—working backward from the anticipated go-live date
- Completion date
- Budgets or costs

This baseline is essential for tracking because it serves as a reference or benchmark which is used to monitor the project's performance. Planning can be compared against the actual results of the project as it begins to take shape. Once a baseline has been established, future changes must undergo the change management process discussed later in this chapter, where all comparisons (variances) are based on the baseline values. Recall the project boundaries—out-of-scope limitations—that need to be documented since they essentially are not funded. The budget requirements and schedule are the project tools and processes most frequently baselined or compared to the start—the scope that contains the requirements.

There are times when leadership, especially on a new project or inexperienced, does not value the time and amount of planning required during this phase in the project's development. But the level of detail needed in the project documents and tools is critical and will ultimately save time later because some important steps were not overlooked potentially leading to project failure. It is important to remember that planning is strongly associated with project success. Again, the primary function of a project plan is to give the PM, team, and organization a road map from the project start to end. The APRN PM will use the key documents noted here as well as those from Chapter 3, Design/Initiation: Project Management—Phase 1, to create this "map." The map must contain sufficient information so that at any point in time the PM knows what remains to be done, when and with what resources the tasks will be completed, and what objectives the project is supposed to meet.

Key Components of a Project Plan: Process and Tools

There are many techniques for developing a project plan, and they are fundamentally similar. You need to develop a systematic analysis to identify and list what must be done in order to achieve the project's objectives, to test and validate the plan, and to deliver it to your stakeholders. This process was started when the needs assessment and gap analysis were completed, which were discussed in Chapter 3, Design/Initiation: Project Management—Phase 1. The key components of the project plan discussed and demonstrated in this chapter are:

- The project plan or resource management plan (work plan), RACI chart, and Gantt chart
- The WBS
- The project schedules, including network diagram and critical path (CP)
- The risk management plan
- The communication plan
- Change management plan
- Status meetings

During the design and planning phases—the first two phases—most of the documents and tools needed during the implementation of the project will be developed. The deliverables (what has to be done in order for the project to progress) and documents needed to start the project include scope and charter, project plan using a Gantt chart, WBS, network diagram, cost estimates, RACI (responsible, accountable, consulted, informed), risk management tool, communication and change management plans, timeline chart, identification and documentation constraints, defining project deliverables, and status meeting processes, documents, and other tracking tools.

As the project moves forward toward implementation, a final step for phase 2 is the Kick-Off meeting, which essentially launches the implementation and energizes the team as they start the next and longest phase of the project—implementation phase. This phase will also add more clarity for the team as they begin to see more structure added to the project as well as clarity to their roles.

PROJECT MANAGEMENT SKILLS AND COMPETENCIES

Leadership foundational skills and knowledge required to lead a project include the *10 Essential Project Management Skills* discussed by Landau (2017). There are many other skills that more experienced PMs may possess but these have been identified as the basic skillset and competencies needed to successfully lead a project to completion. Nurses typically possess many of these skills and knowledge by virtue of practice, albeit at different levels of expertise, but they are also supported further when developing and utilizing the tools identified in this text. The 10 essential skills and knowledge areas include:

- Leadership
- Communication
- Scheduling
- Risk management
- Cost management
- Negotiating
- Critical thinking
- Task management
- Quality management
- Sense of humor

Many of these skills overlap nursing practice in a variety of ways and are not exclusive to project management only but are required for nurse executives, nurse managers, nursing informaticists, and nurse informatics specialists, as well as all nurses, depending on the level of practice and healthcare organization.

Skill development as a PM is supported when developing and using the processes and tools identified in this chapter. For example, the skillset needed for risk management includes the development and utilization of the risk management tool described later in this chapter; the development of communication skills is enhanced during the development of the communication plan.

Barriers to Effective Project Management

According to the Centers for Disease Control and Prevention (CDC, 2011; Box 4.1), there can be a number of problems and barriers to successful project outcomes that teams may face.

BOX 4.1

COMMON BARRIERS TO PROJECT TEAM DEVELOPMENT

Communication problem: When stakeholders are unclear of or possess varying priorities, interests, outlooks, and expectations related to project activities, deliverables, and outcomes

Changes in scope, budget, objectives, regulatory or resource requirements, or other factors

Conflicts among team members resulting from uncertainty in team roles and responsibilities

Competition among team members over positions of authority, power, and/or influence

Lack of a clearly defined and understood team hierarchy, structure, and objectives

Lack of credibility of, or support from, senior management and/or project leaders

Lack of commitment by team members

SOURCE: Centers for Disease Control and Prevention. (2011). *Removing barriers to project team development: Supporting a common project delivery framework.* Retrieved from https://www2.cdc.gov/cdcup/library/newsletter/CDC_UP_Newsletter_v5_i2.pdf

---

Most of the preceding issues can be avoided with detailed planning by developing, tracking, and monitoring documents, requiring accountability for ownership of tasks, carefully managing scope, requiring formal approval of any changes, engaging stakeholders, and emphasizing frequent, effective, clear communication.

> ▶ **QUESTIONS TO CONSIDER BEFORE READING ON**
> 1. What is the difference between a schedule and project plan?
> 2. What is a deliverable?
> 3. What is a WBS? What is its purpose?
> 4. What is an SOW? What is its purpose?

THE PROJECT PLAN

Previously, you may have considered the project plan was a schedule—but they are different. A schedule is part of the project plan that would not succeed without one. The schedule in the project plan defines the due dates for different tasks that need to be completed. There are several types of schedules that will be discussed later. Schedules are critically important in that they can graphically display the project plan and allow a quick overview of the project, owners, and due dates.

One of the first things as the APRN PM is to create a project plan. It is very important to remember that any task started without a plan and due diligence and lack of metrics and/or other specific details is almost always doomed to fail from the start. In the previous chapter, the scope was defined, SMART objectives using the "five Ws and an H" for measurable objectives were developed, and the stakeholders who approved the project were identified. This chapter defines the next steps to developing content, tools, and processes to the project plan.

Deliverables

Preliminary lists of project deliverables are to be created in the scope and charter as described in Chapter 3, Design/Initiation: Project Management—Phase 1. Now that more information is available, you will be able to more clearly define the project deliverables. "Deliverables" are the items needed to meet the goals and objectives of the project. As you did when creating your measurable objectives, add to the project charter dates when these items are due and define how they will be delivered. Remember, the due dates can be adjusted as the schedules are put together. Start by creating the task list of items needed to meet the project deliverables. As the task list is created, add the estimated hours it will take to complete tasks and the owner responsible. The work packages or tasks are unique because each is a deliverable; again, remember that you may need to revise the lists as more information becomes available.

Project Scheduling

One definition of a "schedule"—it is the conversion of a project action plan into an operating timetable where it becomes the basis for monitoring and controlling project activity. This chapter provides a closer look at different types of project schedules needed on the project. Examples are provided to break tasks/work packages from the WBS down into smaller parts or tasks and then organize tasks into the schedule.

First, it is important to understand scheduling terminology and then learn how to take a simple plan and schedule tasks from the WBS manually using network diagrams (Activity Sequencing and Network Diagrams, 2014). Many times organizations provide software, such as Microsoft Project, so that scheduling can be completed more quickly by the PM or designate. The different types of schedules are discussed here, but first an understanding of the WBS used to develop the schedules is needed.

Work Breakdown Structure

The WBS is developed to show the detail of work and specific tasks needed to be completed before the project can be considered ready to implement. However, it is not the project plan or schedule—but a different one. This is one of the first project documents you will need to develop and key to going forward with your project plan. There are a number of different guidelines for describing size of the tasks. The most universal one is to break down the scope into pieces of work assigned an owner.

You must first understand exactly which tasks and activities need to be completed. It helps to see details of the project in smaller, workable, and more manageable components (see Figure 4.1).

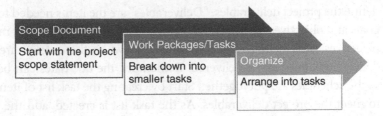

FIGURE 4.1 Steps to developing a work breakdown structure.
SOURCE: Sipes, C. (2016). *Project management for the advanced practice nurse.* New York, NY: Springer Publishing Company.

The WBS is typically completed before the Gantt charts are developed, since it is the first document used to divide the project into smaller tasks. If a task seems too large to manage, that is an indication that it needs to be broken down into smaller activities or, if too small, it can lead to micromanagement of the activity and even conflict in who "owns" the tasks. It provides a quick view for all concerned, including stakeholders, of the project requirements and tasks needed to be accomplished in each of the five phases of the project.

The WBS graphical view shown in Figure 4.2 represents how the work packages or tasks can be broken down into tasks and subtasks. The columns show the WBS code (1; 1.1) and activities.

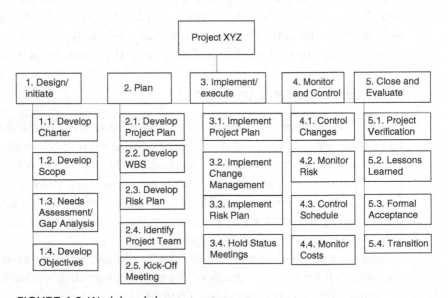

FIGURE 4.2 Work breakdown structure.
SOURCE: Graphical version from Sipes, C. (2016). *Project management for the advanced practice nurse.* New York, NY: Springer Publishing Company.

WBS codes are numbered and indented so that the level of each activity or task is clearly identified. This example represents Project XYZ, which has been funded by a healthcare organization. The figure shows five phases of the project. The five phases of all project management projects are discussed in Chapters 3, Design/Initiation: Project Management—Phase 1, to 7, Closing the Project—Phase 5.

This example in Figure 4.2 is representative of only a few of the tasks needed to complete a project—the one the APRN PM will develop will include much more detail (Chapter 7, Closing the Project—Phase 5).

The tasks for each phase of the project include:

- Phase 1: Design/initiate—four of the tasks to be completed include developing the charter and scope, conducting the needs assessment, and developing the objectives (Chapter 3, Design/Initiation: Project Management—Phase 1).

- Phase 2: Plan—the partial list of the tasks to be completed includes developing the project plan, WBS, risk plans, assigning the project team, and kickoff (Chapter 4, Planning: Project Management—Phase 2).

- Phase 3: Implement/Execute—tasks to be completed include implementing the project, creating the change management and risk plans, and holding the status meetings (Chapter 5, Implementation/Execution—Phase 3).

- Phase 4: Monitor and Control—tasks to be completed include change control, monitoring risk, controlling the schedule, and monitoring costs. It is important to remember that the monitor and control functions overlap the implementation as that is where the processes are originally employed—to monitor and control the implementation (Chapter 6, Monitoring and Controlling: Project Management—Phase 4).

- Phase 5: Close and Evaluate—tasks to be completed include obtaining project verification, conducting a lessons-learned analysis, obtaining final acceptance, and transitioning the project to leadership. The example in Figure 4.2 is representative of only a few of the tasks needed to complete a project—the one the APRN PM will develop will include much more detail (Chapter 7, Closing the Project—Phase 5).

Work Packages/Tasks

After the scope statement has been approved, the team begins to identify work packages/tasks that must be completed to deliver the project's scope. A work package is a deliverable or subset of a project; it can be a miniature project within the large project or a part of the WBS. The work packages are unique because they are each a deliverable; they make work manageable because the APRN PM can detail steps needed to complete each work package. All of the work packages or miniature projects combine to complete the entire project. This allows teams to work on their work packages or deliverables concurrently if necessary.

One of the first steps to identify work packages or tasks is to hold a brainstorming session with the project team. Then tasks identified are collected and documented in the WBS. Using a scope statement, the project is decomposed/broken down into smaller work packages. The end goal is to identify each task at the most granular and detailed level where work can be recognized by the stakeholders. The smaller and more detailed tasks help to facilitate control of the project and improve communication about the project. Finally, after the WBS tasks have been defined with great detail, the next step will be to develop the RACI chart to define duties and responsibilities for all tasks and owners of each task.

Statement of Work

An important note here is if you are working in a larger organization or project management office (PMO), you may be expected to create an SOW but not all organizations require one as there are other documents that contain more detailed information such as the scope and charter. An SOW is a document that outlines the project or service, a timeline for expected completion, deliverables, and assumptions. It also defines how the project should proceed and vendor, if included, expectations and timeline for completion. More frequently today, this information is included in the detail of the scope and charter documents as well as the WBS documents and project plan. In that case the SOW is not needed or redundant if required. Another reason is it is very important to add detail and be very specific when developing all of the project documents and preparing weekly and monthly status reports. This is mentioned here only so that you understand some of the terminology that can be checked further if applicable.

TRACKING SCHEDULES

As you have learned, there are many different types of schedules including the network diagram and critical path. Network diagrams are a "schematic display of the logical relationships" and sequence of activities (Christensen, 2016; Create a Network Diagram—Office Support, 2014; How to customize the network diagram, 2014; Morris, 2014) which provides a quick view of tasks needed to be completed with a particular project. The network diagram enables the APRN PM to determine schedule times for related project activities, critical path of the project, and the float or slack time (the amount of time that an activity may be delayed without delaying the project).

> ▶ **QUESTIONS TO CONSIDER BEFORE READING ON**
>
> 1. What are some reasons to build a network diagram?
> 2. What information is included in a network diagram?
> 3. What information can you obtain from the critical path method (CPM)? How will this be used to plan and track your project?

Why Is It Important to Build a Network Diagram?

One of the most important aspects of project management is building a project schedule. An important tool called a "network diagram" is a great way to track the project tasks, and it provides a quick visual of what needs to be done. There are two good reasons to learn how to develop this tool:

1.   Today most organizations use network diagrams in some form or another.

2.   It is an industry standard.

3.   It provides another great way to track project tasks for what needs to be completed.

There are several ways to build a network diagram; one way will be to use the activity in box (AIB) method (network diagraming) also known as "activity on node" (AON)—they are the same. With this concept, you will be able to determine (a) a project's scheduled completion time, (b) the slack or float time of project activities, and (c) the critical path of your project (e.g., see "Activity Network Diagram (AND): Definition and Example," 2018).

Microsoft Project can make it easy to build a network diagram. It is like adding—you should first do it manually for simple diagrams and critical paths, but when it is more complex use a calculator. Every PM should know how to build a network diagram manually so that he or she really understands the concepts before working in Microsoft Project. The APRN PMs who understand it are much more effective and know how to use the tools more effectively. Those who do not know how to build a schedule manually often make mistakes and negatively impact a project's triple constraints. Practice is required for proficiency. There are also YouTube tutorials to view which you may find very helpful.

To Build a Network Diagram

After the tasks in the WBS are created, they are assigned to the people, or teams of people, who are responsible for delivering the tasks in a step-by-step process. One way to start building a network diagram is to brainstorm with the project team who will record all of the tasks on sticky notes (without regard to sequencing; How to customize the network diagram, 2014). Then start listing tasks in the order they should occur, determine which activities can occur at the same time, and which activities need dependencies—which means one task must be completed before the next can be started (e.g., medical orders must be defined and updated before they can be built). If a task is considered discretionary—that is, it is determined as a best practice or convenience—you may have to wait. However, a subsequent task can begin if the secondary dependency is not completed.

After all tasks have been defined, put notes on a wall after writing in the earlier information and then start to build a network using those notes. If building more complex network diagrams, a second row can be laid out horizontally along with the original row. It is very important to start out simply before moving to a more complex diagram.

Next, activities are assigned to people who will be doing the work—owners. The team will build duration estimates for activities. It is important to work as a team since many tasks are dependent on other activities in the team. The most accurate estimates are built using actual data from previous, similar projects if available. Then activities can be loaded into an automated scheduling tool such as Microsoft Project. At that point, you will be able to determine the project's scheduled completion time, the slack or float of project activities, and critical path of the project. As mentioned, it is also important to be able to build such a network manually; it is better to re-review all concepts after you have done this. See the network diagram and critical path example in Figure 4.3.

The CPM

As you develop the network diagram, you will need to lay out the critical path. The CPM represents tasks or activities that have float or slack of *"zero" days*, which means they cannot be delayed without delaying the entire project—they are critical tasks. Advantages to using the CPM: it defines which tasks must be completed and those that can be done in parallel. It helps to visualize the shortest and longest times to complete the project and where resources are needed as activities are defined along a line showing how they will be sequenced (Baker, 2013; Mind Tools Content Team, n.d.; Ray, 2018; Slate, 2018). CPM can help make a project more successful as detailed activities are more clearly defined and tracked (see Figure 4.3).

Other important terms to understand include:

- AIB—same as a network diagram; it is a graphical representation of the activities that need to be competed
- AON—activity on node; nodes are the boxes, such as "start"
- Early start (ES) = earliest time activity could possibly *start*
- Early finish (EF) = earliest time activity or project could possibly *finish*
- Late start (LS) = latest time activity can *start* and not jeopardize the scheduled completion of the project
- Late finish (LF) = latest time the activity can *finish* without causing the project to be late
- Slack or float for each activity = slack/float is determined by LF – EF or the time between the ES and LS. The slack/float tells you the number of days, weeks, or months an activity can begin late or the number of *extra days, weeks, or months* an activity can take without delaying a succeeding activity or impacting the completion time of the project. Float is the *extra* cushion time built into a project that will not actually cause a delay in the project, so you anticipate which projects might be delayed to some extent.
- *Crashing* the critical path (CP)—adding more resources to activities to get them completed earlier. Caution: *CP* impacts budget and quality—two of your constraints.
- *Fast* tracking—to perform more activities in parallel
- *Resource leveling*—adding resources with related activities to

the same process; this may cause bottlenecks due to resources unavailable for other activities.

■ *PERT (Program Evaluation and Review Technique)*—PERT is a variation on the CPM, a more rigorous approach which uses a statistical formula to calculate time estimates. There are tutorials on YouTube available to develop this skill if the organization requires this scheduling method.

■ *Milestone*—In the network diagram, a milestone is represented by the node or box. These are also the deliverables discussed earlier in this chapter and are listed in the project scope and charter documents discussed in Chapter 3, Design/Initiation: Project Management—Phase 1.

The critical path is the longest path through the diagram in Figure 4.3, which is 16 days—the path and arrows are in gray. The critical path is the longest time tasks on the path can be completed and already has some slack/float built in. Figure 4.3 is representative of only certain tasks and not all on the project, for example, the build of a clinical documentation application. It also shows which tasks must be completed before the next tasks can be started. For example, task 1—if you were conducting a workflow analysis—has to be completed before the medical orders can be developed—tasks 4, 7, 6, and 8—and so on. You need to know what is missing or the *gap* before you can build the medical orders.

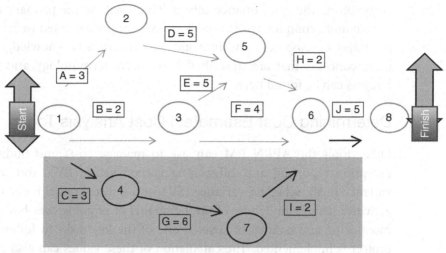

Path 1: A-D-H-J = 3 days + 5 + 2 + 5 = 15 days (1 > 2 > 5 > 6 > 8)

Path 2: B-E-F-J = 2 days + 4 + 5 = 11 days (1 > 3 > 6 > 8)

Path 3: B-E-H-J = 2 days + 5 + 2 + 5 = 14 days (1 > 3 > 5 > 6 > 8)

Path 4: C-G-I-J = 3 days + 6 + 2 + 5 = 16 days (1 > 4 > 7 > 6 > 8)—Critical Path

FIGURE 4.3 Network diagram with critical path.

SOURCE: Sipes, C. (2016). *Project management for the advanced practice nurse.* New York, NY: Springer Publishing Company.

There are many tutorials available on YouTube to practice and polish the skills discussed in this chapter in order to be successful as a PM. You will find these listed in the references section of this chapter.

CSFs for the CPM involve tracking critical tasks and resources; this will determine which tasks affect the project's finish date and whether the project will finish on time.

BUILDING THE BUDGET AND MANAGING THE RESOURCES

Developing the budget is one of the most important tasks the APRN PM will accomplish. Budget management involves the creation and monitoring of a project budget, and identifying, reporting, and escalating variances if they are out of line—moving beyond 5% over the original budget. Tracking costs and resource consumption closely throughout the project is critical and one of the most important tasks a PM will accomplish. The chief finance officer (CFO) will be the primary contact for the more complex budget tasks as PMs are not expected to be experts in budget development and management but must be knowledgeable of basic concepts that are described here. Basic terminology and sample budgets can be found here.

Determining Cost Estimates: Cost Analysis Tools

Other tools the APRN PM can use to manage costs and budgets are exception reporting and calculating earned value (EV). You use cost variance (CV), schedule variance (SV), and indexes to help focus on the activities that are in danger of not being met or of going over budget. The monitoring and control of costs is one of the key tasks to follow as the project is implemented. The calculation of these values can also be done using a software package such as Microsoft Project.

EV Analysis

In order to calculate CV and SV, you will need three very important numbers for each activity. A few important terms to know before beginning to calculate the EV are BCWS, BCWP, and ACWP. The formula is BCWP − ACWP = BCWS or your actual budget. This should not be a negative number, which would indicate being over budget.

- BCWP = budgeted cost of work performed (also called EV)— will change throughout the project
- ACWP = actual cost of work performed—will change throughout the project
- BCWS = budgeted cost of work scheduled

An example of what this might look like:

Table 4.1 shows what a partially completed Gantt chart might look like (originally formatted in Excel).

TABLE 4.1 Gantt Chart

TASK NUMBER	TASK NAME	TASK DURATION	RESOURCE/OWNER	27-OCT	3-NOV	10-NOV	17-NOV
1	**Design project**	**15 days**					
1.1	Hire general contractor	4 days					
1.2	Hire subcontractor	4 days					
1.3	Develop foundation plans	6 days					
2	**Frame and pour foundation**	**25 days**					
2.1	Finish basement prep.	7 days					
2.2	Add drainage around foundation	2 days					

SOURCE: Sipes, C. (2016). *Project management for the advanced practice nurse.* New York, NY: Springer Publishing Company.

The left side of diagram is a tabular structure, with seven rows and eight columns. The column headings are (a) Task Number, (b) Task Name, (c) Task Duration, and (d) Resource/Owner Names to be added. To the right of the Resource/Owner is a graphing area where the duration of the tasks is illustrated with solid lines. The headings in the graphing section are from left to right and are presented in weeks, indicating the estimated length of the task by week—this can also be presented by months.

1. Row 1 = Task Name—**Design Project**. The task bar's left edge starts on Oct 27 and extends to 15 days—bold indicates major tasks; tasks listed under the major task are subtasks.

2. Row 1.1 = Task Name—General contractor. The task bar's left edge starts on Oct 27 and extends 4 days.

3. Row 1.2 = Task Name—Hire subcontractor. The task bar's left edge starts on Oct 27 and extends 4 days.

4. Row 1.3 = Task Name—Develop foundation plans. The task bar's left edge starts on Oct 27 and extends 6 days.

5. Row 2 = Task Name—**Frame and pour foundation**. The task bar's left edge starts on Oct 27 and extends for 25 days.

6. Row 2.1 = Task Name—Finish basement prep. The task bar's left edge starts on Oct 27 and extends for 7 days.

7. Row 2.2 = Task Name—Add drainage around foundation. The task bar's left edge starts on Oct 27 and extends 2 days.

Sample: Preliminary Budget Based on Table 4.1 Information: Planned Budget is:

Design Project—$5,000

- General contractor—$25,000
- Hire subcontractor—$15,000
- Develop foundation plans—**$500**

Frame and pour foundation—$18,000

- Finish basement prep.—$8,000
- Add drainage around foundation—$400

In Week 1, you finalized 40% of the design for the project. In Week 2, you hired the general contractor and revised/updated the project plan and graded the building site. Both of those activities are scheduled to take 4 days. For these exercises, you presume costs are even across time.

BCWS for Week 1 = 40% × $5,000 = $2,000

BCWS for Week 2 = 60% ($5,000) + 25% ($25,000) + 30% ($15,000) + 70% ($500) = $14,100 to get project started

Budget costs accumulate over the life of a project. Therefore, Weeks 1 and 2's costs are added into Week 3's costs and so on.

BCWS for Week 3 = (100% − 60% = 40% due left on designing project) 40% × $5,000 = $2,000 (Total to date: $18,100)

BCWS for Week 4 = 25% × ($15,000) = $3,750 as the subcontractor has asked for an advance on salary

In the example shown in Table 4.2, the actual costs are presented by week. In this case, ACWP is exactly what was budgeted.

TABLE 4.2 Summary of Initial Work Completed

ACTIVITY	WEEK 1	WEEK 2	WEEK 3	WEEK 4
Design project	40%	60%	100%	
Hire general contractor		25%		
Hire subcontractor		30%		25%
Develop foundation plans		20%		
Pour foundation				
Pour basement				
Arrange drainage around foundation				

ACWP for Week 1 = 40% × $5,000 = $2,000

ACWP for Week 2 = 60% ($5,000) + 25% ($25,000) + 30% ($15,000) + 70% ($500) = $14,100 to get project started

Budget costs accumulate over the life of a project. Therefore, Weeks 1 and 2's costs are added into budget costs accumulated over the life of a project, but the percentages in the chart build in that accumulation for you.

ACWP for Week 3 = (100% − 60% = 40% due left on designing project) 40%
    × $5,000 = $2,000 (Total to date: $18,100)
ACWP for Week 4 = 25% × ($15,000) = $3,750

Again, ACWP cannot be calculated until after work begins. In this case you have not calculated how the budget and actual costs are aligned until Week 4 as you are preparing a month-end report for the senior vice president and one of the key stakeholders. This calculation is not difficult; just add up the bills and salaries.

A third calculation is the BCWP. In this case the BCWS + the ACWP + the BCWP are all in agreement. An example of when this might not be the case is when the work scheduled falls behind and more temporary resources are hired to get the project back on track. Then both the *actual* and *budgeted* cost of the work performed would be over budget. BCWP − ACWP should not be a negative number—if so the project is over budget.

Another consideration most companies use is a "loaded rate" to account for pension plans, insurance, and so forth. A loaded rate or a loaded labor rate links variable overhead, fixed overhead costs, and net profit with a unit of labor such as wage or salary. For example, a loaded rate might have an additional 15% to 20% added to cover salary or wages + benefits + overhead costs + profit margin and also include equipment costs and supplies and overhead or operating costs. Some examples might include rent, electricity, gas, water, and sewage. Once you have completed the BCWS, BCWP, and ACWP, the rest of EV analysis is simply plugging in the numbers.

Earned Values

The EV is the budgeted cost of work that has been completed to date of review (current date). EV can also include finished components of a work product. EV is established by the planned costs and the rate at which the team is completing the work to date. Another term is CV, which is the difference between the work that has been completed (in dollars) and how much was spent to accomplish this work. For example: CV = EV − actual cost; another example: CV = BCWP (work performed) − ACWP. A negative result means you are over budget. If you budgeted 20 hours and the actual work was 36 hours = 16 hours were not budgeted.

An SV is the difference between what was planned and what has actually been completed to date. For example: SV = BCWP − BCWS; you have planned that the "Finish basement prep" was going to take 7 days, but it snowed so that the basement prep took 14 days. The budgeted plan of the work performed was only partially completed in the time budgeted—7 days versus 14 days = −7 days over schedule—you are behind schedule because the schedule varied by 7 days.

What to Do About Negative Variances

Being on time and budget are emphasized as doing a great job managing the project. However, if a project is reporting cost and SVs as always too favorable, it could be an indication that work is not being performed with regard to high quality, or efforts have been overestimated. If the project is reporting cost and SVs as too negative, it means something is wrong, or the efforts have been underestimated. The sooner variances are reviewed, the quicker corrective action can be taken. Some projects use variance levels as triggers to alert management to the need for increased oversight. Too much variance in either direction should be closely reviewed. The APRN PM must determine how much oversight is necessary based on the needs of each project, then set these levels and communicate them to all team members and stakeholders.

Estimating Costs

In addition to the methods in Table 4.3, there are several other types of budgeting. Many organizations use a combination of strategies, depending on where they are in the life cycle of a project. It is important for the APRN PM to have basic understanding of some of the terminology.

Fixed costs (Corporatefinanceinstitute, n.d.) are costs that remain constant regardless of the duration of a project or scale of business activity. For example, a purchase of a crane or computer system is the same cost regardless of the duration of the project.

Variable costs (Corporatefinanceinstitute, n.d.) are costs that vary with time or resource changes. For example, labor costs are dependent on the number of hours worked. An example of how you might put the owners/team members and hours each is expected to work on a project is provided in Table 4.3.

TABLE 4.3 Example: Owners/Team Members and Hours Budgeted to Work on Project

RESOURCE NAME			WORK TO DATE			
JOE SMITH			BUDGETED 1,032 HOURS			
TASK NAME	UNITS	WORK (HOURS)	DELAY (HOURS)	START	FINISH	
Analyze workflow	100%	24	0	Mon 10/7/19	Wed 10/9/19	
Team meetings; every 2 weeks	100%	4	0	Thu 10/10/19	Thu 10/17//19	
Start Clinical Doc build	100%	16	0	Thu 10/10/19	Fri 10/11/19	

To Decrease Time: Crash a Budget

"Crashing a budget" refers to a management method for shortening the duration of a project by decreasing the time it takes to complete one or more of the project's activities. In some types of projects, there are standard crash cost formulas that PMs can use to determine how a project's budget would be affected by crashing any activity or activities. Typically the activities reduced are critical activities.

For example, in a clinical documentation project the analyst can use a standard generic application used on other projects or undertake a custom build. In this example, the normal time would be 3 days, with a total normal cost of $300 ($100 per day) to implement the build of the custom application. The crash time would be 1 day to implement the generic application; the total crash cost would be $600. To determine the crash cost difference: 3 days @ $100 day = $300 versus 1 day @ $600 = saving 2 days on the project timeline but $300 over budget. What is the value of doing this? All constraints need to be analyzed for the best approach. This would be an important issue to discuss with leadership including the sponsor. This is a very simple example; most are much more complex but it provides an example of the concept.

CASE SCENARIO 4.1

As you recall from Chapter 3, Design/Initiation: Project Management— Phase 1, Susan, a nurse manager in the cardiac ICU unit, has been assigned to be the PM for a new electronic health record (EHR) system the organization she works for has just approved. She has some management experience but not sure she understands all that is needed as a PM. She is working with the chief nursing informatics officer (CNIO) who has project management experience from previous implementations and she is working with a consultant who has many years of expertise managing new EHR implementations.

The consultant has given Susan a list of "tools" she needs to develop as part of the design of project plan. For Phase 1, Susan developed and completed the:

- Scope and charter
- SOW
- Tasks with metrics
- Due/end dates (timelines) for all phases of the project
- Implementation dates

Now she continues to develop additional tools she will need to track all activities of the project.

Working with the CNIO and consultant, she understands how and why tools are needed. She understands critical tools needed for any project are those she developed for phase 1 and:

- Resource management plan (work plan), RACI chart, and Gantt chart
    - WBS
    - Project schedules, including network diagram and critical path
    - Risk management plan
    - Communication plan
    - Change management plan
- Status meetings' timelines and stakeholders

Susan now puts together a very comprehensive timeline of when all the preceding list of work must be completed in order to set the Kick-Off meeting before implementation—the next phase of the project. She is very nervous

(continued)

as this is a lot of work to accomplish in a short amount of time. She calls a meeting with all of the stakeholders to help put together and finalize the plan, confirm the implementation/go-live dates with schedules now set for 90, 60, and 30 days out from go-live.

1. What should Susan's next tasks be after all dates are confirmed?
2. Who needs the information? What information?

PROJECT RESPONSIBILITY AND ACCOUNTABILITY

Assigning Responsibility

The responsibility assignment matrix (RAM) is an excellent way to clearly assign all of the WBS tasks to a person or another team. The purpose of a RAM document—sometimes referred to as the "RACI"—is to identify who "owns" a specific task or activity as well as the person who is accountable and will sign off on the task when it is completed. To complete the RAM/RACI, first identify all of the project tasks and activities that need to be completed before the project can be implemented. This also includes deliverables and milestones previously identified. Although responsibility can be shared, each activity or task should have only one person responsible as owner, otherwise it may cause issues of ownership. RACI stands for:

- R = Responsible—the person who does the work
- A = Accountable—the person who must ensure that the work is completed (often the PM)
- C = Consulted—this person often has information required to complete the work package
- I = Informed—this is often the largest group and typically includes all of the key stakeholders

As an example of pulling in a few of the tasks from the WBS, Table 4.4 is an excerpt from the project development process outlining who is responsible, accountable, consulted, or informed for specific tasks. It is important to note responsibilities can vary depending on the project. For example, the PM, Joe, generally takes responsibility for the scope and charter documents, whereas in other areas the team selection will require responsibility from Bob, a key stakeholder, but Joe is also accountable.

TABLE 4.4 Responsibility Matrix: RACI

PROJECT TASK/ ACTIVITIES	PM/OWNER OF TASK = R = JOE	APPROVE ACCOUNTABLE/ SIGN-OFF = A = BOB	CONSULTED RE: WORK PRODUCT = C = JIM	INFORMED/ NOTIFIED OF RESULTS = I = SUE
Develop scope	R	A	C	I
Develop charter	R	A	C	I
Team selection	A	R	C	I
Communication plan	R	I	I	I
Risk plan	R	I	I	I
Change control plan	R	I	I	I
Weekly status meetings	R	I	I	I

A, accountable; C, consulted; I, informed; PM, project manager; R, responsible.
SOURCE: Sipes, C. (2016). *Project management for the advanced practice nurse.* New York, NY: Springer Publishing Company.

RISK ASSESSMENT AND MANAGEMENT PLAN

Risk is anything that can negatively or positively impact the project. For example, a positive impact could be a vendor who supplies product before it was expected. This positively impacts the project and helps the project to be completed ahead of schedule. Other risks can negatively impact the project. Not all risks that are identified will occur, but because they can, they must be closely tracked. A risk management plan states how risks will be identified, assessed, and managed during the project life cycle. The APRN PM must be sure that at least the five steps here are completed—there may be more needed but this is the basic process to follow. Next, the risk management plan must be documented with the specific responses to the five steps including:

- Identify risk: internal and external including vendors; list skill levels of all

- Assess risk: prioritize by low, medium, and high

- Manage risk: identify and then either remove or shift it to decrease impact; then re-assess

- Monitor and control each risk: For greater risks, increase frequent monitoring

■ Establish ongoing management plan for risk assessment: requires constant review with weekly reports, more frequent closer to go-live; update and remove risks not impacting project

The process of risk management identifies all positive and negative risks to a project. It is through the risk management plan that the APRN as PM will be able to address and document all risks that could affect the project. Frequent risk reviews keep a focus on risks as they arise and then are managed.

All projects have some risk, especially when more people are involved, which can cause confusion about what needs to be done and when it is due. All risks that could potentially impact the project must be documented and tracked, whether large or small, even though they seem harmless or will hypothetically not impact any other task. This includes all people, processes, technology, environmental influences, and organizational processes. Conducting and updating a risk assessment must be ongoing throughout the entire project. Potential risk areas that must be continually monitored are the all constraints—time, cost/underbudgeted, resources not committed/lacking anticipated skill, as well as:

■ Any budget cuts

■ Role confusion—unclear/undefined responsibilities

■ Lack of stakeholder or leadership support

■ Poor communication

■ Quality of product

These and all other risks will need to be tracked closely on the risk plan shown in Table 4.5.

TABLE 4.5 Sample: Risk Analysis Document and Plan

NO.	RANK	CATEGORY	RISK	DESCRIPTION	TRIGGERS	POTENTIAL RESPONSES	PROBABILITY	IMPACT	RISK OWNER	STATUS/ WAS ISSUE ESCALATED? Y/N
				VERSION				DATE		
	1	Med orders application	High	Not built correctly—does not interface	Nurses documenting med orders	Med orders do not show	High	High	PM, Willow	PM, Willow, IT, in review—Y
	2		High							
	3		Med							
	4		Low							

SOURCE: Sipes, C. (2016). *Project management for the advanced practice nurse.* New York, NY: Springer Publishing Company.

You will need to write down what to do in the event the risk does occur and what to do to minimize and preferably prevent the occurrence.
This entire process must be reviewed with the project team at the weekly
team and stakeholder meetings. Risks that are labeled as "high" should be
addressed immediately as it may delay the forward progress of the project
and potentially lead to failure.

Content for each column can be found in Table 4.5. With each proposed change, it must be logged into the change management log found in
Table 4.6.

TABLE 4.6 Examples of Change Management Log

Project Name: <optional>

National Center: <required>

Project Manager Name: <required>

Project Description: <required>

ID	CURRENT STATUS	PRIORITY	CHANGE REQUEST DESCRIP-TION	ASSIGNED TO OWNER	EXPECTED RESOLUTION DATE	ESCALATION REQUIRED (Y/N)?	ACTION STEPS
	Open	Critical	**EXAMPLE:** Request for product functionality increase			Yes	**EXAMPLE:** Analyze impact of requested change and then meet with the change control board (CCB) to present findings for final decision on the requested change
	Work in progress	High	**EXAMPLE:** The schedule slipped due to unexpected weather-related events			No	**EXAMPLE:** Adjust the schedule to account for the weather-related events
	Closed	Medium					
		Low					

SOURCE: Modified from Centers for Disease Control and Prevention. (n.d.). *Change management log. CDC unified process templates.* Retrieved from https://www2a.cdc.gov/cdcup/library/templates/default.htm

The content in the change management log includes all items that are being changed.

- Rank each risk: highest probability at the top
  - Add source of risk: risk trigger; resolution if triggered
  - Rate: high, medium, and low
  - Impact on project
- Risk owner: who will be responsible if risk occurs?
  - Current status of risk
  - Category: where the risk is in relation to other tasks in the project

CSFs related to risk management include the following:

- Issue is resolved quickly and accurately.
- All issues are documented and tracked with action plans.
- Document of the issue management exists with owners and due dates.
- Communication of key issues is completed and the "who, what, why, where, when, and how" is documented. (Sipes, 2016)

Finally, all risk mitigation plans and success of the plan as well as next steps will be documented. It is important that all risks are quickly identified before they impact project milestones.

COMMUNICATION

Communication is a key aspect throughout a project. All stakeholders must effectively communicate throughout the project's life cycle. A good project plan with poor communication—or a poor project plan with good communication—is ineffective and can lead to project failure. Think of an example of a successful team—football team, other teams, or a team at work. Why are these teams successful or unsuccessful? When comparing the two types of teams, think about the people on the teams. It is not the uniform or equipment but the people. Good communication with the people on the teams is key to project success. Communication is an extremely important skill and key tool for a PM. Knowing who the stakeholders are and making sure you communicate with them effectively and efficiently are a skill common to successful PMs.

Organizations use many different formats when developing a communication plan. Reflect on the formats used at your institution. Communication can take many forms such as written, oral, listening and responding, and observing for nonverbal cues. It is important that communication approaches always include a two-way approach. Some examples are speaking and listening, writing and reading, and sending and receiving messages. Organizational structures can have different communication forms, such as internal, external, vertical, and horizontal. Finally, there are informal and formal communication forms (Change Management Communication Plan, 2018).

Steps that outline how to build a communication plan are listed in Figure 4.4.

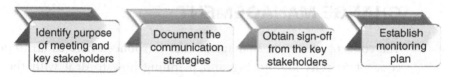

FIGURE 4.4 Steps to developing a communication plan.
SOURCE: Sipes, C. (2016). *Project management for the advanced practice nurse.* New York, NY: Springer Publishing Company.

A documented communication plan and its format is always needed and is an excellent resource for any group of people. If you use the four steps outlined in Figure 4.4, or develop a different one, key to remember is you will develop and use the same communication plan, which will always be consistent in format as people will begin to expect it on a weekly or regular basis.

The project communication plan includes documentation of meetings, status reports, presentations at different steering team meetings such as executive steering team (EST), project steering team (PST), and documentation in a project notebook. It is important to remember your communications must be succinct and to the point. If the EST and other stakeholders are frequently sent unnecessary information, they will stop reading updates, which may be viewed as a waste of time. Something to remember is to focus on getting the right information to the right people at the right time.

It is very important for PMs to be effective communicators. Clear, concise, succinct, and timely communication can add clarity to a complex project. As previously discussed, projects can be matrix, functional, or project structured and, in each case, a PM must be able to effectively communicate across geographic, technical, and business boundaries. From another perspective, a PM with good communication skills can help a failing project. Conversely, a PM with poor communication skills can erode the focus of the project and jeopardize one or more of the constraints.

> ▶ **QUESTIONS TO CONSIDER BEFORE READING ON**
> 1. Why is it important to understand the value of change management?
> 2. What are the 10 principles of change management?
> 3. How would you apply these principles as change is occurring?

CHANGE MANAGEMENT

The concept of change management is introduced here as an important concept to start monitoring and planning how to deal with the many potential issues that may come up as staff and others begin to hear more about the planned change to workflows in the near future. Change management during the implementation phase is more fully discussed in Chapter 5, Implementation/Execution—Phase 3. Change management is difficult because most people do not do it right. According to a 2013 Strategy/Katzenbach Center Survey of global senior executives on culture and change management, "the success rate of major change initiatives is only 54 percent," which is far too low (as cited in Aguirre & Alpern, 2014, p. 3). As PM, you must embrace change as a good thing, keep everyone in the loop, and get necessary approvals on requested changes to move stakeholders and the team to accept changes. The PM and stakeholders' champion must support this effort for it to be successful. There are several ways project change can occur (Aguirre & Rutger, 2013). The project stakeholders may request to change the original approved project scope, or they may want to extend the project schedule, the budget may have been underestimated, and/or the technology was not completely understood, or even a new law or mandate was passed.

Changes to the scope may require a phased approach where portions of the scope are moved to a second or third phase. There are times when the PM must negotiate for more time. The impact of a scheduling change can be far reaching because it affects the budget and many people, including paid contractors and vendors, as well as employees whose commitment to the project has expired. Time extensions are a negative reflection on the PM and should be avoided. Other ways to address any time extensions were discussed earlier, such as analysis of the CPM, with changes that could be made to expedite certain tasks in the project as well as other processes previously discussed.

Some of the most difficult changes occur when there has been an assumption or misunderstanding of what was to occur. If this happens, the easiest approach is to go back and carefully review the list of all of the assumptions, including technology, which should be documented in the scope documents and then reviewed if the assumptions are still relevant. If not they all need to be revised as well as the project schedule, budget, and all other constraints that might be impacted. For change to be effective, it must be clear and determined through collaboration with all stakeholders and decision makers, as well as documented with everyone committed to the change.

The Katzenback Center identified 11 principles for change that they recommend should be used as guidelines when anticipating change.

These include the following:

1. Lead with the culture—determine where the resistance is, how do people behave, and how are decisions made.

2. Engage employees at all levels but start at the top to get support.

3. Involve every layer.

4. Make the rational and emotional case together.

5. Act your way into new thinking—evaluate behaviors, spend time with people to understand thinking and behaviors.

6. Engage, engage, engage, do not just present information in a staff meeting, assign owners to tasks.

7. Lead outside the lines; utilize those recognized as informal leaders.

8. Inspire others, build pride.

9. Leverage formal solutions, reward positive behaviors, provide training that will demonstrate a new functionality or workflow.

10. Leverage informal solutions, be aware of those who would undermine the project.

11. Assess and adapt, be flexible, measure before and after implementing change (as cited in Aguirre & Alpern, 2014, p. 3).

It is critical to assess the mood of an organization. An example where the APRN PM might encounter issues and resistance would be a medical orders implementation or computerized provider order entry (CPOE) in a health system. There are levels of resistance: those who will not learn how to "use a computer" to enter orders so then threaten "blue flu" outages during the go-live, or those who choose not to be involved until the hospital hires scribes to input orders for them. Successful approaches to counter resistance would be to encourage those who are positive about the implementation to be trained as super users and are the "early adopters" and role models.

As nurses, remember the Kübler-Ross process we all learned with death and dying nursing courses. It has been said that staff go through the same phases with change starting with grief of having to give up or change a comfortable habit or workflow used in everyday practice. Lewin's three stages of change management methodology was part of a previous course in most master's programs. The stages were unfreezing, change, and refreezing. During the change stage, it is important to communicate often, dispel rumors, empower action, and involve people in the processes.

The change management process must include setting up a change control board (CCB) where issues and changes are brought forward at least monthly and even more frequently as the project moves closer to implementation. All of the issues, with action plans to resolve the issues, are documented and included in the discussion in status meetings. During the meeting, the project plan is reviewed and discussed, as stakeholders are informed and engaged in decision making. The Change Management Tracking Form can be found in Table 5.4 (see also www.smartsheet.com/free-change-management-templates).

DELIVERABLES AND CSFs

Deliverables

"The term *deliverables* is a project management term that's traditionally used to describe the quantifiable goods or services that must be provided upon the completion of a project. Deliverables can be tangible or intangible in nature." (Investopedia.com, 2019, para. 1). Deliverables were originally identified in the scope document discussed in Chapter 3, Design/Initiation: Project Management—Phase 1, and will be the end product, service, or outcome of the project (see Table 4.7).

TABLE 4.7 Sample: Deliverables for XYZ Project

DELIVERABLE	DESCRIPTION	DUE DATE	OWNER
Scope document	Scope	Oct 10, 2016	PM
Charter	Charter	Oct 10, 2016	PM
Templates for all project documents	Communication, Risk, RACI plans, and all other documents	Oct 10, 2016	PM
Budget	Budget	Oct 10, 2016	PM; CFO

CFO, chief financial officer; PM, project manager; RACI, responsible, accountable, consulted, informed.

SOURCE: Sipes, C. (2016). *Project management for the advanced practice nurse.* New York, NY: Springer Publishing Company.

Critical Success Factors

Rockart (1979) was one of the first to define CSFs as the limited number of areas in which results, if they are satisfactory, will ensure successful competitive performance for the organization. "There are the few key areas where 'things must go right' for the business to flourish. If results in these areas are not adequate, the organization's efforts for the period will be less than desired" (Rockart, 1979, p. 1). CSFs are those elements that are critical to a project success (see Table 4.8).

TABLE 4.8 Sample: CSFs for XYZ Project by Priority

1. Status reports—appropriate people informed (stakeholders and sponsors; status is documented timely weekly, biweekly with due dates and task owners; next steps
2. Scope document updated—after approved by stakeholders—communicated to all associated with project
3. Budget—project budget is within 5% of original approved budget; projections are reasonable and realistic; approved by stakeholders
4. Charter is updated with all scope changes, approved by key stakeholders and management, and communicated to all
5. Governance—end user buy-in and involvement documented; owners identified, responsible, accountable, timely decision documents with due dates—making sure all issues and risks resolved timely, and project completed on time and on budget

CSF, critical success factors.

O'Reilly (2018) further defines the five CSFs (2014) as follows: executive sponsorship who may be the funding sources or the project will impact their departments; project management champions who support the project in a number of ways; prioritizing and defining problems early; identifying ways to fix the problem; and stakeholder engagement discussed earlier.

IMPORTANCE OF STATUS MEETINGS

Status reports are critical because they provide the timely status of the project at least on a weekly basis to all involved in the project including stakeholders. The reports provide updates to the planning and implementation process and establish a formal pattern of the way to keep everyone informed. These status meetings should be set up at the beginning of the project. They can be set up in Outlook as recurring over the duration of the project and should include everyone who needs to know and be kept in the loop regarding the status of the project. The meetings occur for 1 hour at least on a weekly basis, frequently set weekly at 90 days prior to go-live, then much more frequently at 60 days, and then daily 30 days before go-live, unless there are issues with the project.

Tips for Successful Status Meetings

The status meeting must follow the schedule established and documented in the communication plan. The APRN PM must know the status of the project before this meeting. Information is gathered by collecting data from each team member and any others who are involved in the project with assessment of each task; look for progress, backlogs, or barriers to the project moving forward; reflect on key points; and speak to key team members and all task owners to gain their perspectives. The purpose of the meeting is to keep everyone informed on the status of the project but also to do the following:

- Keep the project moving in the right direction
- Help any new team members assimilate into the team
- Help the team work together—there can be team building activities during the meeting
- Provide time to discuss and address any issues that have arisen between meetings
- Provide time for the PM to coach and mentor the team members
- If there are key issues—that is, the project has yellow or red status, invite key leadership to discuss resolution or how to escalate issues

During the first meeting, review the ground rules for meetings, such as the following:

- No cell phones
- Meeting starts on time and ends on time
- Discussions not germane to the topics for the current meeting will be put on the parking lot to be discussed later
- No rabbit trails or war stories
- No side bars
- No "heat-seeking" missiles—verbally discrediting some team member
- One speaker at a time
- Establish trust, value all input

Remember organization, confidence, and respect can be contagious. The PM must be organized and decisive, such as developing a standard status meeting format and meeting agendas. The PM must respect the team members, their time constraints, and also be confident in their roles. This sets the stage for the leadership role and model of the APRN as PM, which can spread through the team. In order to keep the team focused and moving, remember, even if complex and potentially negative issues are handled or discussed in the meeting, the PM should always close the meeting on a positive note. Provide positive feedback to the team, encourage and motivate them, and reach out to each member. Applaud the accomplishments to date as well as the ongoing progress. Stress the tremendous teamwork that goes into deliverables about to go-live. Always leave the team with the notion they are part of a team going to complete a successful project by working together, respecting and supporting one another.

Finally, by way of review, the eight steps to a successful meeting include:

1. Plan the meeting
2. Develop an agenda
3. Set expectations explained before meeting starts
4. Conduct the meeting
5. Always review the next steps before adjourning the meeting
6. Discuss benefits and concerns the team may have
7. Debrief the meeting—what went well, lessons learned
8. Prepare and distribute minutes within 48 hours of the meeting that include a plan of action

KICK-OFF MEETING

A Kick-Off meeting is held when the project has been approved just prior to the next phase—the implementation of the project. All project stakeholders, sponsors, administrators, and team members should be included as well as the vendors. The goal of the Kick-Off meeting is to ensure that everyone is on the same page before the project moves forward to be implemented. It is an opportunity to motivate the team and stakeholders.

Information that will be presented in the meeting includes:

- Goals and objectives of project
- Scope
- Process to request any changes
- Assumptions and constraints
- Risk management plan
- Communication plan
- Each team member's roles and responsibilities
- Schedule and work plan milestones; set at 90, 60, and 30 days prior to go-live
- Key sponsors and stakeholders

This meeting is also a way to validate the project plan, emphasize the importance of the project, and introduce concepts and team members to leadership and other interested parties. It also sets the expectations, guidelines, and timelines for the project as well as introduces project sponsors and key stakeholders to the group. It emphasizes the need that everyone on the team be on the same page.

Prepare the PowerPoint Presentation for the Kick-Off Meeting

The first step is to schedule the meeting and include everyone who is affiliated with the project so that they can hear the same message at the same time. It will be important to communicate using all of the methods previously discussed in case someone cannot physically attend the meeting but can access it through conference call, webinars, Skype, or other means, especially if some members are remote.

Next develop the agenda for the meeting and list the invitees. At the onset of the meeting, take attendance. Ask key stakeholders and sponsors for input into the agenda prior to sending it out. Schedule the meeting for 1 hour allowing time at the end for questions and comments, usually 10 minutes. Send meeting materials out well in advance of the meeting, add it to calendars if Outlook or some other means of scheduling is available, post it in a public place, and then send follow-up reminders the day before the meeting. In addition to earlier lists sent, the agenda should include the following:

- Date, time, and location including conference call numbers and pass codes
- List of attendees and key contact information for the PM (the PM will have other contact information and should act as the conduit for information)
- Welcome to meeting
- Project plan with itemized list of topics that will be covered, the deliverables and due dates
- Review of roles and responsibilities for each team member
- Include a next-steps discussion; finalize any decisions that were not clear, if possible
- Include specific timeline of what tasks happen and when they are due
- End with the Q & A session

Send the agenda and other handouts to all attendees including handouts of the PowerPoint presentation. Encourage invitees to bring questions after they have reviewed the project plan and provide comments where relevant.

On the day of the meeting, test all communication methods to make sure they have been set up and are functioning properly. Check to make sure the meeting room is set up and equipment is functioning for the PowerPoint presentation. At the start of the meeting, introduce the key stakeholders and sponsors as well as other key invitees—introduce team members. It is always a good idea to invite the stakeholders and/or sponsors to say a few words but ask them prior to the meeting if they would like to say a few words—do not surprise them during the meeting. These administrators should be positive about the success of the project with an emphasis on this project having priority over other work. The RACI has already been developed; further contract information can be added to that document and then provided as a handout during the meeting.

Review all key CSFs—these should be key success factors that are specific to the project. It is frustrating when people speak in generalities and do not address the current project. Stay focused and specific. Review the project plan—tasks, responsibilities, milestones, key issues, project dependencies, and risks. This review helps to establish the plan. Remember to review all plans that have been developed, including the resource management plan, communication, procurement, and other project documents.

Finally, during the Q & A session, the PM always tries to thoroughly answer all questions and welcomes input. If questions cannot be fully answered, make sure to let the person know when you will get back with the answer. Typically, the APRN PM should have the answers as well as create an atmosphere where team members know the expectations and a culture that respects the work being done as well as demands high-quality work that meets scheduled deadlines.

CRITICAL THINKING QUESTIONS AND ACTIVITIES

Change management concepts were introduced in this chapter.

1. What are some areas of resistance to change you have observed?
2. Consider how you would address these issues of resistance. How would you implement change in your organization? Develop a plan and discuss it with your team.

SUMMARY

This chapter covered some of the most important concepts and principles of project management as the APRN PM begins to apply the concepts to a project while the tools needed to track and manage the project during implementation are developed. The APRN PM also has learned to develop new tools that will be needed to closely track the progress of the project. Resource management is critical to the success of a project. Having a schedule is critical to successful resource management. Therefore, it is important to understand how to create a schedule. One tool that can be used is a network diagram. The project's activities were assigned to people with expertise in a specific area who will be doing the work. They build duration estimates for the activities. The most accurate estimates were built from previous experience with similar projects. This allowed the determination of a project's scheduled completion time, the slack or float of project activities, and the critical path of your project. The change management process was introduced as well as tips to running a successful status meeting including the final Kick-Off just before project implementation.

REFERENCES

Activity Network Diagram (AND): Definition and example. (2018). Retrieved from https://study.com/academy/lesson/activity-network-diagram-and-definition-example.html

Activity Sequencing and Network Diagrams. (2014). Retrieved from https://www.education.psu.edu/geog584/l5_p4.html

Aguirre, D., & Alpern, M. (2014). *10 principles of leading change management.* Retrieved from https://www.strategy-business.com/article/00255?gko=6c601

Aguirre, D., & Rutger, V. P. (2013). *Culture and change management survey.* Retrieved from https://www.strategy-business.com

Baker, S. (2013). *Critical path method (CPM).* Retrieved from https://h5pm.sph.www.sc.edu/courses/J716/CPM/CPM.html

Centers for Disease Control and Prevention. (2011). *Removing barriers to project team development: Supporting a common project delivery framework.* Retrieved from https://www2.cdc.gov/cdcup/library/newsletter/CDC_UP_Newsletter_v5_i2.pdf

Change Management Communications Plan. (2018). Retrieved from https://www.smartsheet.com/free-change-management-templates

Christensen, E. (2016) *What your boss would like to know about project network diagrams* [Blog post]. Retrieved from https://www.lucidchart.com/blog/what-your-boss-would-like-to-know-about-project-network-diagrams

Create a Network Diagram—Office Support. (2014). Retrieved from https://support.office.com/en-us/article/Create-a-Network-Diagram-A3E8CC62-27C5-4E94-AAAB-6FBC470B6D33

Critical Success Factors. (2014). *Identifying the things that really matter for success.* http://www.washington.edu/research/rapid/resources/toolsTemplate/art_success_factors.pdf

How to customize the network diagram; view in Microsoft Project. (2014). Retrieved from http://www.projectknowledge.net

Investopedia.com. (2019). Deliverables. Retrieved from http://www.investopedia.com/terms/d/deliverables.asp

Landau, P. (2017). *10 essential project management skills.* [Blog post]. Retrieved from https://www.projectmanager.com/blog/project-management-skills

Mind Tools Content Team. (n.d.). Critical path analysis and PERT charts. Retrieved from http://www.mindtools.com/critpath.html

Morris, R. (2014). *The network diagram.* Retrieved from http://www.netplaces.com/project-management

O'Reilly, G. (2018). *5 critical success factors for project management improvement* [Blog post]. Retrieved from https://www.brightwork.com/blog/5-critical-success-factors-for-project-management-improvement

Ray, S. (2018). *Understanding critical path in project management* [Blog post]. Retrieved from https://www.projectmanager.com/blog/understanding-critical-path-project-management

Rockart, J. (1979). Chief executives define their own data needs. *Harvard Business Review, 57*(2), 81–93. Retrieved from https://hbr.org/1979/03/chief-executives-define-their-own-data-needs

Sipes, C. (2016). *Project management for the advanced practice nurse.* New York, NY: Springer Publishing Company.

Slate, A. (2018). *Critical path method: A project management essential.* Retrieved from https://www.wrike.com/blog/critical-path-is-easy-as-123

ADDITIONAL READING

Communication: The message is clear [White Paper]. (2013). Retrieved from http://www.pmi.org/business-solutions/white-papers/communication-clear-message

Ferrier, J. A. (2014). Project management in health and community services: Getting ideas to work, 2nd edition [Book review]. *Australian Journal of Primary Health*, *20*(1), 122. doi:10.1071/PYv20n1_BR2

Franklin Covey Co. (2012). Franklin Covey Co. launches project management essentials for the unofficial project manager: Anyone can be a successful project manager. *Business Wire*. Retrieved from https://www.businesswire.com/news/home/20121212005223/en/Franklin-Covey-Launches-Project-Management-Essentials-Unofficial

Heldman, K. (2013). *PMP: Project management professional*. New York, NY: Wiley.

Ho, J. (2010). Project management in health informatics. *Studies in Health Technology & Informatics: Health Informatics, 151*, 413–424. doi:10.3233/978-1-60750-476-4-413

CHAPTER 5

IMPLEMENTATION/ EXECUTION—PHASE 3

LEARNING OBJECTIVES

Upon completion of this chapter, the reader will be able to:

1. Define the implementation phase.

2. Discuss three tasks to be accomplished during the implementation phase.

3. Discuss the value of a change management plan.

4. Discuss three steps to develop the change management plan.

5. Discuss why it is important to engage stakeholders.

6. Discuss why it is important to define and monitor critical success factors (CSFs).

OUTLINE

- Key Terms
- Introduction
- Overview of Project Implementation
- Implementing Project Management Plans

- Implementation Checklist
- Managing Project Teams: Leadership Skills
- Managing Project Stakeholders
- Status Meetings
- Change Management in the Implementation Phase
- Minimizing Scope Changes and Scope Creep
- Communication Plan in the Implementation Phase
- Testing
- Summary

KEY TERMS

- Execute
- Implementation
- Lewin's change theory
- Metrics
- Phases/steps of project management
- Stakeholders
- Testing

INTRODUCTION

The next step in project management is the implementation, which corresponds to the implementation phase of the nursing process. Project implementation "requires that everyone involved, including the members of the unit staff understand the goal, expectations, and timeline. A well-run project allows all participants to be able to instantly access the data. Success depends on every team member being a part of the implementation process in ways that are vital and change oriented. Every team member is responsible for investigating why mistakes made will contribute to the process change" (Overgaard, 2010, p. 53).

Nursing and project management go well together and overlap in many processes. As discussed earlier, project management includes project initiation, planning, implementation, monitoring, and closing. "Originally conceived as a tool to ensure that projects using many disciplines would be correctly budgeted and completed within a scheduled time frame, project management has become useful in a variety of settings from writing a book to building a skyscraper. The use of the systematic steps in project management can eliminate costly mistakes, increase quality, and save time" (Whole Building Design Guide Project Management Committee, 2017, p. 1). As discussed in Chapter 2, Advanced Practice Nurse Role Descriptions and Application of Project Management Concepts, correlations to the nursing process were demonstrated and may help the nurse manager understand how using a systematic process to complete a project is beneficial.

In this step, phase 3 of project management, the project will be implemented or executed as some organizations refer to it. You will begin to apply the tools that were discussed and developed in the previous phases. The project activities such as applying the concepts of monitor and control will help you step into the role of a project manager (PM). In this phase of project management, tool implementation developed in the previous phases—design and planning—will be implemented.

> ▶ **QUESTIONS TO CONSIDER BEFORE READING ON**
>
> 1. Of the different phases of project management, which one is implementation?
> 2. Discuss how the phases of project management correlate to the nursing process.
> 3. What are the primary objectives of the implementation phase?
> 4. What activities are included when utilizing the tool kit?

OVERVIEW OF PROJECT IMPLEMENTATION

In the previous phases, you learned that there are five standard phases to a project: design/initiation, planning, implementation/execution, monitor and control, and closing the project, where evaluation and lessons learned are conducted. Some organizations have combined steps and refer to only four steps in the process, while others may break the steps out further and refer to six steps in the project management process. Whichever process best fits the project or activity, it is important to remember that you may use all of the steps or only a few. It is important to remember, too, that a "project" is only a temporary activity, such as planning a wedding or developing a project for a graduate practicum, just as the steps in developing a patient care plan can be a temporary activity.

Five Standard Project Management Phases: Similar to the Nursing Process

The five standard project management phases or stages are very similar to the nursing processes and are described here.

Design/Initiation

The design/initiation process establishes the feasibility and goals of the project. It is during this phase that the project is authorized. Many times there is some confusion regarding the project management terminology that is used by an organization. Frequently both terms are used—design and initiation—at the first phase where the project starts to come together with thoughts and ideas of what should happen in the project. In this first phase, the project charter and scope documents are developed; these documents help provide direction to the project.

Planning

Project constraints are referred to as the "triple constraints of cost, quality, and schedule," but more frequently today, many more have been identified that need closer monitoring, such as risk, methods used, who the customers are, skilled resources, scope of project, the organization, and sustainability of the project. The project plan will need to address all of the constraints (Benz, 2018). This is the phase where all activities or the work related to the project is defined as well as a schedule is developed for the project. The project plan and tool kit should include the goals, deliverables, schedule, communication strategy, risk management, work breakdown structure (WBS), network diagram, budget, and a human resources plan such as a Gantt chart with owners responsible for each task with due/end dates identified. Stakeholders need to be identified at this point. The work is now planned and will be implemented as the tools that were developed in this second phase of the project management are applied. The phase ends with the kick-off meeting.

Implementation/Execution

Here again, many times different terminology is used to mean the same thing depending on the organization. More frequently today, the term "project implementation" is used to mean this is the third phase of project management—where implementation of the plan utilizing all of the tools happens, including adding resources such as the team members and "products" and functionality that were previously tested and built. This is when the plan that was developed in the previous phases of project management is implemented, where the content from both the scope and charter documents, as well as all of the tools such as the risk, change management, communication, and other documents, is used to track and monitor progress toward achieving the final outcome—the deliverables. Status meetings have been established and implemented as part of the communication plan as has the human resources plan that includes how the team will develop and be nurtured, as well as specific assignments and responsibilities that will need to be completed. The communication plan has been finalized for the stakeholders, and the risk management plan is implemented.

Monitor and Control

The monitor and control processes are ongoing throughout the entire project; any issues need to be quickly addressed. Change requests will be monitored very closely—there may even be denial of changes, or changes may need to be moved to a different time or phase such as optimization for implementation—depending on the total project impact. This is when the status of the project is monitored against the schedule. A key question to ask is "Are the steps when controlling and monitoring the schedule specific enough to indicate on time, at or under budget, and the production of quality products with minimal risk?" Are all preceding constraints addressed and monitored and controlled?

Closing and Evaluation

Typically, the last phase of project management is closing and evaluating the project. It entails resolving any issues and completion of all necessary final documents and reports for terminating the project. The team will debrief and compile useful information, such as lessons learned concerning the completed project for current and future reference of what worked well and what would need improvement before utilizing the same process and tools again. The information will then be presented to the stakeholders in a final PowerPoint presentation where the PM will receive final verification and sign-off from leadership. At this time, the team is also disbanded and moved to another project or back to previous work.

IMPLEMENTING PROJECT MANAGEMENT PLANS

Primary Objectives

The main objective as the project is implemented is to apply the concepts, tools, and methods discussed in the previous chapters that will support the ongoing management of the project. The outcome of the project will be a "deliverable" that meets the requirements of the organization. The primary objectives when implementing a project are:

- Apply a standardized method and steps in an organized way so that creation of the project deliverable is completed in an orderly way and that steps or important elements of the project are not overlooked. It is very important to remember that if you do not have the time to do it right the first time, when would you find time and money to do it over? The art of being consistent is also very important to team members as it provides stability rather than constant change.

- It is important to be trustworthy and as transparent as possible with the team members and stakeholders so they can anticipate the next steps in the project development.

- Learn to be a good decision maker—be timely and goal orientated, and consult team and stakeholders when necessary. Provide project updates daily or weekly on whatever process was established as you developed the project plan. If there are requests for more information, revise the communication plan to meet the needs of both the team and stakeholders.

- Remember to monitor the constraints that have been identified as critical to the project, which includes, but are not limited to, being on budget and on time as well as others previously discussed when delivering the business objectives of the project.

- If resources do not have a specific commitment to this project, monitor them closely as they may be shared with other projects or have other time commitments, which can be confusing for all and even delay the project if they are not available as originally planned.

Implementing/Executing the Project

Review the details of the implementation/execution phase with the team and stakeholders. Make sure that there is a thorough understanding of the plan by all so it can be monitored to keep the project and everyone moving in the right direction. Have the timeline posted where everyone can see it and update as needed. Key to timely implementation is to start from the kick-off meeting and work backward from the due date of the planned implementation. Mark the timeline for Day 90, Day 60, Day 30, and Day 0 with colorful tags so everyone is aware of the key strategic points to go-live. Remember to build and nurture the teams as well as to manage the project and communicate, communicate, and communicate in a variety of ways to make sure everyone is in the loop.

▶ **QUESTIONS TO CONSIDER BEFORE READING ON**

1. What happens during an implementation?
2. Who is involved during an implementation?
3. What is the purpose of the change control board (CCB)?
4. What is the difference between leaders and managers?

IMPLEMENTATION CHECKLIST

The project management methodology has been discussed, and the tools needed to monitor and control the implementation were developed in phase 2—planning step. The next step is to apply both the processes and tools. The main components of implementation include those found in Table 5.1.

TABLE 5.1 Implementation Checklist

STEPS	ACTIVITY	RESPONSIBILITY	DUE DATE
1	Maintain updated project plan and evaluation	Project manager	
2	Monitor tasks and document next steps	Project manager	
3	Manage issues and escalate as necessary	Project manager; project team, stakeholders	
4	Manage and report risks	Project manager; project team, stakeholders	
5	Develop CPM and monitor	Project manger	
6	Manage budget	Project manager; stakeholders	
7	Manage project communications and presentations	Project manager; project team	
8	Manage meetings—team, stakeholders, other executives	Project manager; project team, stakeholders	
9	Manage and create timely status reports	Project manager	
10	Document, document, document	Project manager; project team	
11	Evaluate need for education and training	Project manager; project team	

CPM, critical path method.

SOURCE: Sipes, C. (2016). *Project management for the advanced practice nurse*. New York, NY: Springer Publishing Company.

It is best to keep a copy of the checklist available to check off tasks in progress and/or completed at least on a weekly basis.

CASE SCENARIO 5.1

As you recall from Chapter 3, Design/Initiation: Project Management—Phase 1, Susan, a nurse manager on the cardiac ICU unit, has been assigned to be the PM for a new electronic health record (EHR) system the organization she works for has just approved. She has some management experience, but she is not sure she understands all that is needed as a PM. She is working with the chief nursing informatics officer (CNIO) who has project management experience from previous implementations, and she is also working with a consultant who has many years of expertise managing new EHR implementations.

(continued)

From Chapter 4, Planning: Project Management—Phase 2, Susan developed the tools she will need for the implementation of the project. She developed and completed the following:

- Scope and charter
- Statement of work (SOW)
- Tasks with metrics
- Due/end dates (timelines) for all phases of the project
- Implementation dates

In this phase, implementation, she has developed and received sign-off from the key stakeholders. She also developed the following additional tools:

- Resource management plan (work plan), responsible, accountable, consulted, informed (RACI) chart, and Gantt chart
- WBS
- Project schedules, including network diagram and critical path
- Risk management plan
- Communication plan
- Change management plan
- Status meetings timelines and stakeholders

After all of the design and planning has been completed, teams are assembled as the go-live date is 5 days away.

1. Susan has arranged the go-live meeting for all teams. What are Susan's next steps?

   a. What are the key documents she needs to review with all teams?

   b. Who needs to be included and responsible for managing issues?

      i. Where would she find this information?

   c. What is the role of the CCB?

   d. Going forward, what are the CSFs that need to be monitored? Where and to whom would this information be reported?

Application of Tool Kit to Maintain Updated Project Plan

The main objective is to review and track the work plan on a regular basis to determine how the project is progressing in terms of schedule, budget, scope, risks, and issues. Basic objectives to accomplish this are to monitor and document the progress from the beginning of the project to avoid surprises. Revise the plan for accuracy as needed, then communicate to the team and stakeholders; if changes are required, they will need to go to the CCB that has been established for review and approval. Has new work been identified that may have been overlooked? Review the project milestones—are they on schedule? Are they being impacted by other tasks not previously considered?

Other monitor and control activities include reviewing and documenting tasks that have been completed and then updating the plan to reflect this. Determine what resources were used, the cost, and if they impacted the current plan in any way. Review the plan to assess if any tasks have been delayed, and determine the cause by conducting a root-cause analysis as well as a review of any and all other tasks that might be impacted.

As the plan is updated, review the due/end dates again to make sure the project is on time, and conduct a critical path analysis from Chapter 4, Planning: Project Management—Phase 2, using the critical path method (CPM) example discussed in the planning phase, which defines tasks that cannot be delayed without delaying the entire project. Work with team members and stakeholders to determine ways to accelerate tasks to get back on track, including working overtime or adding more resources.

With plan updates, it is important to include the team members, to remain transparent, and include all communication with the team and other stakeholders. Managing the implementation noted in Table 5.1 means to:

- Conduct a review and analysis of all dates, status, descriptions of the tasks, and resolution of issues and the owner.

- Review next steps with the team and stakeholders to make sure they are accurate.

- Document any changes required, and also send the updated plan to the CCB for review, approval, and sign-off if needed.

- Identify and review with the team any work that is not currently in the plan called "scope creep."

- Review if and how it will impact the project, that is, if you delay the project by days or weeks.

- Will it impact another task or subtask?
- What is the cost and risk?
- Any delay in a milestone will need to be evaluated by leadership, executives, and stakeholders to determine the impact on the entire project. An evaluation of the project to either crash it or push it to meet deadlines will be reviewed and decisions made. Review crashing and fast-tracking a project in Chapter 4, Planning: Project Management—Phase 2.

In summary, CSFs to implementing a project include monitoring that all tasks are completed effectively, on time, and within budget—the "triple constraints" as well as all others—such as risk, methods used, who the customers are, skilled resources, scope of project, the organization, and sustainability of the project as identified by Benz (2018). Monitoring that all team members maintain responsibility for the tasks assigned to them and there are no task delays due to lack of completion is also critical. Finally, monitor that all risks have been identified, mitigated, and there are no remaining unresolvable CSF tasks. This phase—implementation—is where the tool kit, functions, documents, and concepts are applied. The potential need to revise and update any tools and documents and then reapply them to the project is an important step to close monitoring and controlling of the project.

MANAGING PROJECT TEAMS: LEADERSHIP SKILLS

You may take responsibility for the leadership role as PM with a project team working with you, depending on the size of project you are working on, enterprise wide or a much smaller project. Or it could be one of the project management roles as part of the graduate practicum experience working with a mentor. One important aspect of management is to understand the difference between a manager and a leader. You will have an opportunity, or may have had in the past, to research and study a number of leadership theories, such as transformational leadership, and how to apply them, but that is not the purpose here. The purpose of this text is to reflect on a process, steps, discipline of project management, and what to do as manager of a project and define how it all applies to developing leadership knowledge and skillsets based on the theoretical foundations.

Nurses have functioned in management roles for many decades—this is not a new concept. Historically, Florence Nightingale was both a manager and a leader (Gardner, 1993; Huxley, 1975). She managed, changed, and revolutionized the health system in the British military in the mid-19th century. You may become or are familiar with many leadership theories previously discussed that define the skills used and that are inherent to good leaders.

You may have shadowed a mentor or other manager during a practicum experience. Have you had a chance to reflect on how management and leadership overlap? As an advanced practice nurse (APRN), today's expectations are to accept and undertake more leadership roles. Gardner's work is considered foundational, as he has conducted a number of research studies on leadership. According to Gardner (1993; Gardner & Avolio, 1998), leadership and management overlap in many ways and "[m]ost managers exhibit some leadership skills, and most leaders ... find themselves managing" (1993, pp. 6). Azad et al. (2017) argue that leadership and management are the same thing while others argue that leadership and management are not the same thing, but they overlap. The specifics of management tasks are compared in the list of tasks leaders perform (see Table 5.2).

TABLE 5.2 Overlap Between Leaders and Managers

LEADERS	MANAGERS
Set goals	Set goals
Plan	Plan
Set priorities	Set priorities
Keep system functioning by setting agendas	Keep system functioning by setting agendas
Make decisions	Make decisions

SOURCE: Adapted by Sipes (2016) from Gardner, J. W. (1993). *On leadership.* New York, NY: The Free Press. Retrieved from http://www.altfeldinc.com/pdfs/JohnWGardner.pdf

As you work with others on the project team, think about how and what you are doing fits as either a manager, leader, or both. As a new manager, you have learned a number of skills in the graduate program. You have had the opportunity to apply those skills and experience the outcomes of the skills and tasks completed while developing more skills as a PM.

REFLECTION QUESTIONS

How are the functional activities as a PM different because you also have a theatrical background, deeper learning in graduate courses, and other qualities you bring as a nurse leader to the project team?

Reflect on the opportunities you have had to interact and empower different team members, your mentor, and even other leaders.

■ What are some key attributes you will take from these experiences?

Reflect on what you will and will not do in the future as you incorporate the concepts of project management into the role and define the type of leader you are or aspire to be.

Other qualities important as a leader and manager are also defined as "project management attributes." These include the importance of motivating team members, planning and priority setting, organizing, allocating resources, agenda setting, and decision making. Azad et al. (2017) further discuss "the two terms 'leading' and 'managing' form the framework for skills and abilities that are necessary for an individual to drive team success. In fact, the concepts of leadership and management are transposable, especially in describing performance effectiveness within organizations" (p. 102). Do these attributes sound like those discussed previously as project management skills?

As Gardner noted in 1993, and still fundamental concepts relevant today, leadership skills include:

■ Motivating: Effective leaders tap those that serve the purposes of collective action in pursuit of shared goals. They accomplish the alignment of individual and group goals. They create a climate in which there is pride in making significant contributions to shared goals.

■ Managing: Leadership and management are not the same thing, but they overlap. It makes sense to include managing in the list of tasks leaders perform.

■ Someone has to plan and set priorities.

■ Someone has to design the structures and processes through which substantial endeavors get accomplished over time.

- Someone has to keep the system functioning, mobilizing, and allocating resources; directing, delegating, and coordinating; reporting, evaluating, and holding accountable.
- Someone has to set agendas and make decisions (1993, p. 6).

It is important to reflect on pressures frequently encountered as a "leader." According to Gardner, Avolio, Luthans, May, and Walumba (2005), "we are told that people look for organizational leaders of character and integrity to provide direction and help them find meaning in their work" (p. 344). Leaders who model ethical behaviors expect others to follow and practice by example.

> ▶ QUESTIONS TO CONSIDER BEFORE READING ON
> 1. Who are stakeholders?
> 2. What are the roles of the stakeholders in a project?
> 3. How do you communicate with stakeholders?

MANAGING PROJECT STAKEHOLDERS

Stakeholders who were identified in the design and planning phases have, by definition, a vested interest in the project and need to be kept informed of the project status. They need to be identified and the buy-in and support obtained early then maintained throughout the project. The importance of and how to conduct the stakeholder analysis is discussed in Chapter 3, Design/Initiation: Project Management—Phase 1. Some stakeholders have little interest in the project but need to be kept informed, while others "own" many aspects of the project, which will impact their operations. It is important to respect their time so it will be important to prepare a succinct status report for all stakeholders. The resources that have an interest in the project were identified earlier—now you will need to prepare a status report for this phase of the project for them.

Stakeholder Presentations

You will need to communicate to determine what the stockholders expect in the way of status reports, be it weekly, biweekly, or only on a monthly basis. It is important to obtain a signature/sign-off for each report presented as a means to track the communication trail. The reports must be succinct with the most important details only and to-the-point to demonstrate respect for everyone's time; so prepare only key points. If more information is requested it can be provided later. In the report, include:

- An introduction of key stakeholders and roles in the organization
- Project objectives—how these are being met
- Project issues
- Project barriers—will these delay the project; what are costs associated with these?
- Next steps with owners
- Due dates

The goal of the stakeholder reports is to get approval and acceptance for the progress made on the project and to keep them informed of all steps in the project progress. It is important to remember, these are very important people who have an interest in and support for the project. If this is a graduate practicum project for both master's and doctoral programs, and you are working with a mentor, the stakeholder group helped to identify the project needs and deliverables as well as provided funding for the project. A stakeholder can also be an end user who had input into how the project should be designed and then implemented. If there are a number of end users, it is best to have one or two representatives of the group in attendance at these presentations. If there are too many attendees with opposing views of how the project should be designed and implemented, it can delay the project further and prevent closing of the project in a timely manner or even project failure due to indecision.

The one thing to remember is change will be constant throughout the project and therefore needs to be constantly monitored, controlled, documented, and reported to all involved. The monitor and control documents and examples are discussed in Chapter 6, Monitoring and Controlling: Project Management—Phase 4. They should be used throughout the project to identify changes that need to be made, then presented to the CCB and all stakeholders. By now you have discovered how the many different processes must be constantly monitored and controlled. Good project management also depends on the project team and performance against the 10 constraints of time, cost, and scope and others discussed earlier (Benz, 2018).

Key ongoing tasks that should be monitored and controlled for possible revisions and updates include:

- Project plan
- Project objectives
- Project milestones and timeline
- Project performance metrics
- Project issues and risks
- Project change control
- Project team performance

Reflect on the key tasks critical to constantly monitor but may not be the reason why projects fail. Do you see the potential correlation between the two—failure to monitor and control—one leads to failure of the other? What process will you use to do this? How will you document the process? Where and to whom will you present the information?

STATUS MEETINGS

Status meetings and status reports were discussed in Chapter 4, Planning: Project Management—Phase 2. One of the most important tasks a PM must undertake is to communicate, communicate, and communicate effectively with all team members and leadership. One critical component is to plan and hold effective and productive meetings as previously discussed. An effective and productive meeting can also enhance decision making for the project. It is important to set goals and objectives for the meeting to provide a framework for effective decision making. This is now where the application of what was previously planned is implemented. There are seven key steps to conducting an effective meeting. See Table 5.3 for content needed in status reports. By way of review, these are:

1. Plan the meeting.
2. Always have an agenda; create the agenda with goals, objectives, and times; have the various owners present reports and updates; distribute before the meeting.
3. Conduct the meeting; start and stop on time; review ground rules; no rabbit trails; document conversations/minutes; document participants.

4. Review next steps; assign owners to different tasks and document with due dates.

5. Document benefits and concerns (B & Cs); there are no wrong answers.

6. Summarize—what went well, what could have gone better, and lessons learned.

7. Write up, record decisions, next meeting date, and distribute minutes within 48 hours of meeting; one-page summary with attachments if necessary.

CSFs presented for any meeting must include informing leadership of issues and progress so there are no surprises. Team members are kept up to date on project activities, status, and the decision-making process. Finally, decisions regarding any changes are made and approved within the critical time frames defined.

TABLE 5.3 Weekly Project Status Report

Project Name:	Week Ending:
Project ID:	Project Manager:
Description of Project:	Project Start Date:
Project End Date:	% Complete:
Project Issues:	Causes:
Project Risks:	Proposed Mitigation:
Project Is On Time, On Budget, Within Scope Green (OK) Yellow (In trouble—Watch) Red (In danger—Escalate)	
Sign-off: Project Manager: Stakeholder: CEO/Other Leadership:	

SOURCE: Sipes, C. (2016). *Project management for the advanced practice nurse.* New York, NY: Springer Publishing Company.

CHANGE MANAGEMENT IN THE IMPLEMENTATION PHASE

Concepts of change management and documentation processes were introduced in Chapter 4, Planning: Project Management—Phase 2, as this is where the processes should be initiated and tracked. "Sometimes the problem is not outright conflict but an unwillingness to cooperate. One of the gravest problems George Washington faced as a general was that the former colonies, though they had no doubt they were all on the same side, were not always sure they wanted to cooperate" (Gardner, 1993, p. 7).

Change Management Tracking Tool

The concept of a CCB has been discussed several times. Most organizations have a CCB or change management team that usually meets at least once a month, 90 days before a project is implemented, and then biweekly 1 to 3 months before implementation/go-live, as more issues arise at that time due to a variety of reasons including various levels of testing. Principles of monitor and control for project changes include informing all involved stakeholders to get approval for all proposed scope changes, which must be signed-off before they can be implemented. *All* change requests must be evaluated against impact on other elements of this and other projects currently in development. *All* project changes are communicated to *all* team members and stakeholders. Changes are evaluated against how they will impact an application, functionality, or process in another part of the organization or throughout the entire enterprise.

In the implementation phase, it is important to understand the processes and rationale behind change theory, and why an understanding of what happens is important to the changes that will occur during implementation. If implementing a project for a graduate practicum as an APRN, the one thing to learn with progression through the practicum is that change is constant. Monitor and control documents must be developed and then be used to identify changes that need to be made and presented to the CCB. See Table 5.4 for the example of information needed in a change request form. In addition to the example in Table 5.4, you need to add columns for: Impact Summary, Change Request Type, Date Identified, Entered By, Actual Resolution Date, and Final Resolution and Rationale, for example, CCB approved.

TABLE 5.4 Change Request Form

IDENTIFICATION OF CHANGE	DATA
Change Request	Change request number; date received; date revised; project number, name, requester name, department
Requestor Information	Describe change, reason, priority
Change Information	Impact on stakeholders, organization
Status Information	Next steps: owner, date, decision, due date
CCB Approvals	Signatures

CCB, change control board.
SOURCE: Sipes, C. (2016). *Project management for the advanced practice nurse.* New York, NY: Springer Publishing Company.

Ten principles for change were discussed in Chapter 4, Planning: Project Management—Phase 2, as well as an example of a change management log, which should help understanding.

Change management theories help to better understand what change is, why people are impacted by the inconsistency, feelings of loss of control caused by change, and how to address change management in nursing practice. Important to remember is that nurses deal with change every day and use change, information, and knowledge to make sound practice judgments. Just as nursing science informs nursing and the nursing process, project management concepts focus on the integration and use of project management processes and tools, which can improve management of patient care issues. Understanding change by exploring change and diffusion of innovation theories helps to identify and explain behaviors that may be seen before changes occur. Supporting the impact of change and all involved ultimately provides for quality patient care outcomes.

Diffusion of Innovation Theory

The two theories important to explore are diffusion of innovation theory and change theory. The diffusion of innovation theory explores behaviors and concepts of those who lead opinions, those who follow, and how the media can influence the opinion leaders as well as the opinion followers. The theory describes the process that people go through to adopt something new, such as a product, idea, practice, philosophy, or other theory. The theory is very important in project management because new things are introduced, and this theory helps to understand the diffusion or process through which the innovation is or is not adopted.

REFLECTION QUESTIONS—DIFFUSION OF INNOVATION AND CHANGE THEORIES

- When you read Kaminski's (2011a, 2011b) diffusion of innovation information on change, reflect on a change that you experienced in relation to some point in the project management process up to this point.
    - As you learned new ideas, how did that occur—through practice or other?
    - Can you relate it to the diffusion of innovation theory?
- Change theory is another important theory by Lewin. Change theory describes a three-phase process in which we open our minds, deal with the change, and adopt the change. It is important to understand the dynamics when dealing with change and expecting others to deal with change also.
    - Think about different reactions to the change.

(continued)

(continued)

> ■ Can you trace the phases as described by Lewin and apply those to differ-
> ent behaviors you see during a change event?

Lewin's Change Theory

There are many rules for management of change and to decide when to execute it to be very effective. Managing organizational change will be more successful if applying these simple principles. Achieving personal change will be more successful too when using the same approach where relevant. Change management requires thoughtful planning and sensitive implementation and, above all, consultation with and involvement of all of the people affected by the changes.

If change is forced on people, expect problems to arise. Change must be realistic, achievable, and measurable. These aspects are especially relevant to managing personal change. Before starting any organizational change, ask:

■ What do we want to achieve with this change?

■ Why?

■ How will we know that the change has been achieved?

■ Who is affected by this change, and how will they react to it?

■ How much of this change *can* be achieved ourselves?

■ What parts of the change need help?

These aspects also relate strongly to the management of personal as well as organizational change.

In summary, understanding and application of nursing theories can be critical to the success and ability to implement effective systems designed to improve patient care. Reflect on the theories used in nursing practice and their applications including if in a graduate practicum. Reflect on behaviors of others and how you felt as controls and familiar systems and workflows changed in your practice.

MINIMIZING SCOPE CHANGES AND SCOPE CREEP

Minimizing scope changes must be continually assessed in order to prevent scope creep. Possible reasons for unplanned scope changes can be many including overlooking a needed component or functionality, business changes and upgrades needed now rather than later, and many other factors or even a request from a provider to "just do this little thing for me"—not realizing the downstream impact that change might have on the entire enterprise systems statewide (Sipes, personal communications, 2016).

To better understand what might cause changes in the scope plan, you need to understand the potential reasons that might cause the project to change. Some of these reasons might be related to the following:

- A shift in business focus

- Change in timeline

- Change in budget and funding sources

- Change in key sponsor, stakeholder, and other leadership commitment

- Change in technology requirements, upgrades, and new vendor products

- Unclear definition of overall project requirements and support where requirements are not aligned with overall organizational scope

All of the areas listed here need to be fully evaluated by the PM and project team and then reported to stakeholders and leadership to define, evaluate, and develop a plan for mitigation of the changes.

COMMUNICATION PLAN IN THE IMPLEMENTATION PHASE

Types of Communication

Communication as a skill was discussed in Chapter 4, Planning: Project Management—Phase 2. During the implementation phase, a communication plan will need to be developed and communicated to the project team and all invested in the project. When developing the communication plan for the project and team, it is important to consider different types or ways of communicating effectively. It is important to remember that people have different learning styles; therefore, creating a communication style that fits the different learning styles will go a long way to effective communication (Ray, 2017). A summary of the types of communication are listed in Table 5.5. Can you think of other important ways to get a message out?

TABLE 5.5 Communication Plan

TYPE OF INFORMATION	PARTICIPANTS	PURPOSE	FREQUENCY	TRANSMITTAL	PREPARED BY
Status Meetings	Project team sponsor	Report project status, including significant accomplishments, issues, and costs	Distributed prior to the scheduled meeting	Email Meeting	Project manager
Change Requests	Program staff Project sponsor Project manager	Communicate, receive approval, and document status of all change requests	As needed	Email Meeting	Project manager
Project Plan	Project team	To articulate project background, scope, roles/responsibilities, risk, deliverables, schedule, staffing, communication, and closeout	At project start-up	Email	Project manager
Kick-Off Meeting	Project team	The kick-off meeting is used to clarify goals and objectives, individual roles and responsibilities, and interdependencies	Once at project start-up	Meeting	Project manager Meeting
Weekly Status Meeting	Project team	Discuss status, issues, and concerns related to the project	Weekly	Oral presentation Discussions	Project manager

SOURCE: Adapted from Ray, S. (2017). *What is a project management communication plan?* [Blog post]. Retrieved from https://www.projectmanager.com/blog/project-management-communication-plan

Communication Mistakes

Being a good communicator takes skill, practice, and continual effort. Good communication is difficult and is an art. Have you ever sent off a message or written a document that has numerous typos and spelling errors? Or have you read a document or email from someone else full of errors or assumptions of what you may or may not know? What was your impression of that person? Have you ever attended a meeting where there was no direction or agenda? How did that make you feel? Disorganized? At what point is it best to have face-to-face meetings?

Another frequently cited error is delivering bad news via email, which must be done in a personal, face-to-face communication, or, even worse, by forwarding others' emails that were not intended for others to see, potentially violating and creating privacy and security issues.

A mistake new PMs frequently make is to assume everyone understands exactly what is being said. In this case it is important to ask for questions and use multiple approaches to getting your message out. Never assume that your messages are always understood. Always have an open mind to other effective ways of completing a task or suggestion.

TESTING

One of the most important functions a PM can oversee and manage is that of testing of the deliverables. Unfortunately, when there is a time crunch on a project, testing is the one function that is cut back or eliminated. It is also one of the biggest reasons projects might fail. You may have experienced this or remember the issues with the healthcare system or a smaller project rollout.

Why Is Testing Important?

As this concept is so important, it is discussed again in Chapter 6, Monitoring and Controlling: Project Management—Phase 4. As a review, Cable News Network (CNN) reported, "An internal government memo written just days before the start of open enrollment for Obamacare warned of a 'high' security risk because of a lack of testing of the HealthCare.gov website" (Johns, 2013, para. 1). Additional comments from CNN, "officials of companies hired to create the HealthCare.gov website cited a lack of testing on the full system and last-minute changes by the federal agency overseeing the online enrollment system" (Cohen, 2013, para. 2).

Testing is typically broken down into five phases:

1. Individual programming modules/unit testing
2. Component/compared against requirements
3. Integration
4. System as a whole
5. User acceptance testing (UAT) or beta testing

Systems are designed by application or module; each module or application is first tested individually. Depending on the testing process, the individual applications or modules are gradually integrated and then tested. Finally, all of the applications that have been tested and passed are moved into the entire system where they are then tested as a whole.

Acceptance, beta testing—also known as "UAT"—is the final phase before implementation of a system and refers to whole system testing, corrections made, with the final step as implementation. Here end users are asked to test the system to see if it meets their specific workflow, are all task applications included, and is the system easily navigable. If involved or you have an opportunity to view the testing processes, the opportunity will provide valuable information and insight into the project management process and lead to understanding of how critical the testing phase is.

You may also hear the term "usability testing." Nine key principles of usability, listed by Healthcare Information Management Systems Society (HIMSS, 2018), are simplicity—it is easy to use, natural, consistent, efficient, forgiveness and feedback, effective use of language—terminology, effective information presentation, minimize cognitive load, and preservation of context (HIMSS, 2018, p. 1). It is important to understand how this fits with testing as these are many of the elements incorporated into test scripts that are used by testers/end users to test the system. An HIMSS survey (2009) reports that one reason EHR adoption and implementation rates have been very slow is due to lack of efficiency and usability of current systems.

Overall, projects have failed when the importance of testing was put aside and not done due to time constraints—the Obama healthcare rollout is just one example of the consequences when the value and importance of testing are ignored. Can you think of any other examples where a project failed due to lack of testing?

CRITICAL THINKING QUESTIONS AND ACTIVITIES

1. Consider that your organization is about to change things with the installation of a new EHR. What will you do to address resistance by staff to change?

    a. Put a plan in place to address this—where would you start?

2. The system has been unit tested. At what point would you get the end users involved in testing?

    a. You will need to develop a test script for the end users—nurses from the ICU.

What content would you include as you develop the test script? (You can find examples of how to do this at: https://usersnap.com/blog/user-acceptance-testing-example.)

SUMMARY

This chapter provided the tools and concepts used in the implementation phase, the third phase of project management. In this phase tools that were previously developed in the design and planning phases were implemented, and processes were tracked, monitored, and controlled. Leadership skills were discussed as well as change management theories with suggestions on how to manage change and different behaviors that might be seen during this phase. Finally, critical thinking questions and activities were presented as a means to add to the expertise leaders and mangers will need to develop and apply in leadership roles.

REFERENCES

Azad, N., Anderson, H. G., Jr., Brooks, A., Garza, O., O'Neil, C., Stutz, M. M., & Sobotka, J. L. (2017). Leadership and management are one and the same. *American Journal of Pharmaceutical Education, 81*(6), 102. doi:10.5688/ajpe816102

Benz, M. (2018). *10 project constraints that endanger your project's success* [Blog post]. Retrieved from https://www.projectmanager.com/blog/10-project-constraints-that-endanger-your-projects-success

Cohen, T. (2013). Contractors blame government for Obamacare website woes. *CNN.* Retrieved from https://www.cnn.com/2013/10/24/politics/congress-obamacare-website/index.html

Gardner, J. W. (1993). *On leadership.* New York, NY: The Free Press. Retrieved from http://www.altfeldinc.com/pdfs/JohnWGardner.pdf

Gardner, W. L., & Avolio, B. J. (1998). The charismatic relationship: A dramaturgical perspective. *Academy of Management Review, 23,* 32–58. doi:10.5465/amr.1998 .192958

Gardner, W. L., Avolio, B. J., Luthans, F., May, D. R., & Walumba, F. O. (2005). Can you see the real me? A self-based model of authentic leader and follower development. *The Leadership Quarterly, 16*(3), 343–372. doi:10.1016/j.leaqua.2005.03.003

Healthcare Information Management Systems Society. (2009). *A call for action: Enabling healthcare reform using information technology.* Retrieved from https://www.himss.org/sites/himssorg/files/HIMSSorg/2009CalltoAction/ HIMSSCallToActionDec2008.pdf

Healthcare Information Management Systems Society. (2018). *HIMSS EMR usability evaluation guide for clinicians' practices: 9 essential principles of software usability.* Retrieved from https://www.himss.org/himss-emr-usability-evaluation-guide-clinicians -practices-9-essential-principles-software-usability

Huxley, E. J. (1975). *Florence nightingale.* New York, NY: Putnam.

Johns, J. (2013). Goverment memo warned of high security risk at health care website. *CNN.* Retrieved from https://www.cnn.com/2013/10/30/politics/obamacare-website -warning-memo/index.html

Kaminski, J. (2011a). Theory applied to informatics: Lewin's change theory [Editorial]. *Canadian Journal of Nursing Informatics, 6*(1). Retrieved from http://cjni.net/ journal/?p=1210

Kaminski, J. (2011b). Theory in nursing informatics column: Diffusion of innovation theory. *Canadian Journal of Nursing Informatics, 6*(2). Retrieved from http://cjni.net/ journal/?p=1444

Overgaard, P. (2010). Get the keys to successful project management. *Nursing Management, 41*(6), 53–54. doi:10.1097/01.NUMA.0000381744.25529.e8

Ray, S. (2017). What is a project management communication plan? [Blog post]. Retrieved from https://www.projectmanager.com/blog/project-management-commu nication-plan

Sipes, C. (2016). *Project management for the advanced practice nurse.* New York, NY: Springer Publishing Company.

Whole Building Design Guide Project Management Committee (WBDG). (2017). *Project planning, delivery, and controls.* Retrieved from https://www.wbdg.org/about -wbdg-whole-building-design-guide

CHAPTER 6

MONITORING AND CONTROLLING: PROJECT MANAGEMENT—PHASE 4

CAROLYN SIPES | TRACY STOGNER

LEARNING OBJECTIVES

Upon completion of this chapter, the reader will be able to:

1. Define three components of the monitor and control phase.

2. Discuss three tasks to be accomplished during the monitor and control phase.

3. Discuss the value of monitoring and controlling a project.

4. Discuss when the monitor and control functions should be implemented.

5. Discuss three reasons projects fail.

6. Discuss the 80/20 rule.

7. Discuss one method to monitor the quality of a project.

8. Discuss the continuous quality improvement (CQI) process.

9. Discuss the role of evidence-based practice (EBP) in quality improvement.

OUTLINE

- Key Terms
- Introduction
- Overview of Monitoring and Controlling a Project
- Implementation of the Monitor and Control Plan
- Quality Control
- Benefits and Process of Change Control
- Quality Control: Useful Processes and Tools for Problem Solving
- Testing
- Summary

KEY TERMS

- 80/20 rule
- Continuous quality improvement (CQI)
- Critical success factors (CSFs)
- Deming's plan, do, check, act (PDCA) cycle
- Donabedian's model
- Evidence-based practice (EBP)
- Failure mode effect analysis (FMEA)
- Key performance indicators (KPIs)
- Lean Six Sigma
- Milestones
- Pareto principle
- Root cause analysis (RCA)
- Strengths, weaknesses, opportunities, threats (SWOT) analysis

INTRODUCTION

The monitor and control process is about managing the juggling act the project manager (PM) must master during the project implementation process. In Chapter 5, Implementation/Execution—Phase 3, the discussion centered on how to implement a project when using different processes and tools. This chapter covers the "who, what, why, where, when, and how" to conduct the ongoing project management (Sipes, 2016).

With implementation comes monitoring and controlling that must occur throughout a project. Monitoring and controlling project processes ensures the project team is completing its work correctly and according to the project plan. It might feel like trying to manage the universe at times: time, money, teams, product, communication, quality, and the list goes on. All of these elements must be monitored and controlled in order to have a successful project. This is where the PM must keep everything flowing and truly manage scope, time, costs, risk, quality, and other constraints discussed in earlier chapters. Using the tools developed in the design and planning phases will provide the guidelines and framework needed to manage the project.

Finally, as you continue to manage the project, there is a need to continually evaluate the project progress against the original goals and objectives you initially developed for this project, as well as the mission statement, timeline, and project plan.

▶ **QUESTIONS TO CONSIDER BEFORE READING ON**

1. What is the primary objective of monitor and control processes?
2. What are some of the activities associated with monitor and control processes?

OVERVIEW OF MONITORING AND CONTROLLING A PROJECT

Standard Processes

The monitor and control process of a project requires frequent checking to make sure all tasks are applied in a standardized way, that there is frequent communication about the project status, effective decisions are made toward achieving the goals, and deliverables identified in the scope meet due dates as well as quality standards. Finally, it is important to determine resources continually meet requirements for completing the project in a standardized way.

IMPLEMENTATION OF THE MONITOR AND CONTROL PLAN

Primary Objectives

Key to monitoring the project at this phase is to review the project plan on a regular basis—at least weekly at 90 days from go-live and then more frequently at 60 and 30 days from go-live—to determine how the project is moving forward in terms of time, due dates, budget, scope, issues, and risks.

Other objectives that greatly impact projects require they be monitored from the very beginning of implementation to avoid surprises. If there are problems, evaluate and revise the plan to make sure all activity can be monitored and tracked. Be sure all new work not currently in the project plan has been identified and assigned an owner. Evaluate the project milestones and due dates to determine if dates are being met. If there is an issue, consider conducting a critical path analysis and/or ways to crash the project. These processes and details on how to accomplish this were discussed in Chapter 4, Planning: Project Management—Phase 2.

Activities

All activities should be closely monitored and included on the timeline as well as identification of activities previously completed so the project plan can be updated and resources reassigned if necessary. Always track and report percentage completed in the weekly status reports, especially information that goes to leadership and stakeholders. The weekly status report tool and process is available in Chapter 5, Implementation/Execution—Phase 3. Closely review all activities to make sure all dependencies are completed; be sure to indicate and list which activities and how they might impact other activities if not accomplished. After completing this assessment, be sure to document and update the project plan and then send new, updated copies to all stakeholders.

If the plan needs to be revised, obtain needed information by requesting feedback from every team member, then hold a status meeting so that all team members can determine if and how changes might impact their tasks. Include all team members in the decisions and determination of next steps as well as updated due dates if indicated. Finally, communicate, communicate, and communicate to set expectations for all involved in the project, including stakeholders and leadership. Also document objectives, expectations, problems, milestones, and critical success factors (CSFs).

New Work

If new work that is needed to complete the project has been identified during the monitoring and controlling process, pull the team together, and have everyone participate to determine who "owns" the new work, the due dates, and if it really is part of another task or should be moved to the next phase. Review to understand if the new work is associated with a milestone. If not, establish one, and document it in the work plan. You can find budget tracking tools, as well as the application and processes used, in Chapter 4, Planning: Project Management—Phase 2.

Budget

During implementation, it is necessary to track the budget very closely to determine how much of the budget has actually been used based on tasks completed and then determine how much money is left when conducting the budget analysis. Also review to determine where future large expenses might occur so that these can be planned accordingly. It is important to get weekly reports back from team members during the status meetings to determine how much work remains so you can determine costs or the need for approval of additional budget items.

> ► **QUESTIONS TO CONSIDER BEFORE READING ON**
> 1. What are some reasons projects fail?
> 2. What are important tasks that need to be monitored during this phase?
> 3. What is the 80/20 rule?
> 4. How is the 80/20 rule applied?

QUALITY CONTROL

Benefits and Process of Monitor and Control: Why Projects Fail

As previously discussed, there are many different processes that must constantly be monitored and controlled. Good project management depends on the project team and their performance against constraints—time, cost, quality, risks, and scope as well as others previously identified. It is important to reflect on how well the process is going with frequent discussions of how to do things a bit differently going forward if problems arise. There are many reasons why projects might fail. Here are a few key reasons to keep in mind:

- Someone on the team wanted to help out an end user by just "tweaking" an application and thought there would be no impact on the system, but in fact it took the system down, leading to delays and cost overruns.

- Scope creep—doing "favors" for end users or stakeholders, adding additional tasks that are outside of the budget.

- Lack of good communication with the team and among leadership. For example, the stakeholder thought the project was to solve problem XXX when the direction of the project is going YYY.

One way to help mitigate the risk of failure is to constantly reconfirm any plan against the project plan, objectives, the scope, and charter documents. Good, ongoing communication is critical, not only with the project team but also with leadership and stakeholders who have an interest in and are committed to this project.

Key ongoing tasks that should be monitored, if not daily at 30 days prior to go-live but at least three to four times a week, include the following:

- Project plan—all components
- Project objectives
- Project milestones and timeline
- Project performance metrics
- Project issues and risks
- Project change and quality control
- Project team performance

When monitor and control documents were created and then applied to the project, were there questions overlooked or not considered, such as the following?

- Who will be accountable, in addition to you, the PM? List others in the leadership role.

- What is the potential impact on the live system if the change is implemented?

- What is the potential impact on the go-live date, if any?

- What would postlive maintenance requirements be?

- What would potential impact on your budget be?
- How will change, if approved, impact the overall scope of project?
- What is the quality of the tasks performed when pushed too quickly against a deadline?

There are many reasons why projects can fail. Table 6.1 summarizes this well and provides some of the more common and frequently seen risks (Carlos, 2018).

TABLE 6.1 Reasons Why Projects Fail

PROBLEM	CAUSE	RISK
Poorly managed	Undefined objectives and goals	Lack of management commitment
Lack of a solid project plan	Lack of user input	Lack of organizational support
Centralized proactive management initiatives to combat project risk	Enterprise management of budget resources	Provides universal templates and documentation
Poorly defined roles and responsibilities	Inadequate or vague requirements	Stakeholder conflict
Team weaknesses	Unrealistic time frames and tasks	Competing priorities
Poor communication	Insufficient resources (funding and personnel)	Business politics
Overruns of schedule and cost	Estimates for cost and schedule are erroneous	Lack of prioritization and project management
Scope creep	No change control process	Meeting end-user expectations
Ignoring project warning signs	Inadequate testing processes	Bad decisions

SOURCE: Adapted from Carlos, T. (2018). *Reasons why projects fail.* Retrieved from https://www.projectsmart.co.uk/reasons-why-projects-fail.php

The Pareto Principle

As noted in Table 6.1, there are many reasons why projects fail—both simple and complex; the list is only a partial list. One way to look at this is to focus on most common reasons a project might fail using the Pareto principle. This principle is called the 80/20 rule, meaning that the most common reasons a project might fail can be that 20% of the defects cause 80% of the problems; therefore, a good rule is to focus 80% of your time on the 20% of the work that is really important (Reh, 2018). If the items and tasks listed in Table 6.1 are closely monitored, there is a good chance there will be few issues—this process of monitoring but not understanding lessons learned from previous projects is a much needed and a huge benefit of the monitor and control process.

Summary of Tools to Monitor and Control

Table 6.2 summarizes the tools and chapters where found, which correlate with the phases of the project life cycle where the documents would be developed. By way of review, each chapter also includes a discussion of the application processes.

As previously discussed, the documents needed to monitor and control the project were designed and planned in previous phases and then applied during the implementation phase as the process of monitor and control is also initiated. It is very important that all tasks are monitored; if not using the documents provided, it will be important to at least develop some way to track and monitor all items during the implementation phases.

TABLE 6.2 Summary of Tools Needed to Monitor and Control With Location

PROCESS	TOOL	CHAPTER WHERE FOUND
Scope	Scope tool	3
Charter	Charter tool	3
Project timeline	Example	3
Gap analysis	Example	3
Stakeholder analysis	Stakeholder analysis tool	3
SMART objectives	SMART objective tool	3
WBS	WBS tool	4
SOW	No tool	4
CPM	CPM tool	4
Tracking—network diagram	Network diagram tool	4
Budget	Budget tool	4
Risk	Risk tool	4
Change management	Change-tracking log	4
Weekly status meetings	Meeting tool	4
Project deliverables	Deliverables tool	4

(continued)

TABLE 6.2 Summary of Tools Needed to Monitor and Control With Location (*continued*)

PROCESS	TOOL	CHAPTER WHERE FOUND
Kick-off meeting	PowerPoint presentation	4
RACI	RACI tool	4
Implementation checklist	Checklist tool	5
Status report	Report tool	5
Change request	Change request tool	5
Communication plan	Communication plan tool	5

CPM, critical path method; RACI, responsible, accountable consulted, informed; SOW, statement of work; WBS, work breakdown structure.

SOURCE: Sipes, C. (2016). *Project management for the advanced practice nurse.* New York, NY: Springer Publishing Company.

PROCESS OF CHANGE CONTROL

No one likes change. As discussed in Chapter 4, Planning: Project Management—Phase 2, many resist change at all costs, especially if it is a big change such as the implementation of the electronic health record (EHR). With the implementation of a large project such as an EHR, it will change many things including workflows, where to find things, and how to complete a task. Smaller changes such as evaluation of an improvement process from a single project a doctor of nursing practice (DNP) completed may not see as much resistance to the new ideas and change as in other projects. Depending on the change, there typically is resistance, and the larger the change, the more there is resistance. During large EHR implementations, there may even be resignations as people do not want to learn new processes or tasks or even feel threatened that their lower-level skills will be exposed. An example of the change-tracking log can be found in Chapter 4, Planning: Project Management—Phase 2; the change request form can be found in Chapter 5, Implementation/Execution—Phase 3.

> ▶ **QUESTIONS TO CONSIDER BEFORE READING ON**
> 1. What is the purpose of the plan, do, check, act (PDCA) cycle?
> 2. What is involved in CQI?
> 3. Who was Donabedian?

QUALITY CONTROL: USEFUL PROCESSES AND TOOLS FOR PROBLEM SOLVING

The process of plan, do, check, act (PDCA) is a familiar process used when assessing and tracking project tasks and deliverables. Historically, Deming in the 1950s proposed that "business processes should be analyzed and measured to identify sources of variations that cause products to deviate from customer requirements" (Arveson, 1998, para. 1). He recommended that business processes be placed in a continuous feedback loop so that managers can identify and change the parts of the process that need improvements.

Although the quality control process of analyzing the root causes was developed for businesses and industry including engineering, the process is viewed as providing a standardized means of monitoring projects of any size. The PDCA defined here has four tasks commonly applied; some organizations may vary the process to only three tasks—PDA—plan, do, act. The PDCA acronym is:

- **PLAN**: Design or revise business process components to improve results.
- **DO**: Implement the plan and measure its performance.
- **CHECK**: Assess the measurements, and report the results to decision makers.
- **ACT**: Decide on changes needed to improve the process.

Deming's PDCA cycle (Figure 6.1) reflects a continuous, ongoing cycle. Monitoring the implementation of any project will benefit from an ongoing and continuous evaluation of how the different aspects are being implemented, where there may be gaps in the process, implementing corrections, and then rechecking the process again (Table 6.3).

Quality management or control requires that tasks be continually monitored such as using a continuous quality improvement (CQI) process and all project documents updated with information sent to all team members and stakeholders—everyone who has a part in the project. It includes such components as budgets, costs, project plan, scope document, testing, metrics, changes and change control, and risks to name a few. A more comprehensive list is included in Table 6.1. It is important to remember that project documents are "living documents," which means they need to be monitored closely and updated as needed, with review and approval from the change control board (CCB) as indicated.

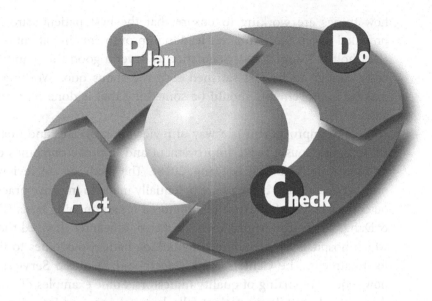

FIGURE 6.1 Deming's PDCA cycle: continuous, ongoing cycle.
SOURCE: Courtesy of Karn G. Bulsuk.

TABLE 6.3 PDCA Tool

Plan	Identify the problem, and conduct a gap analysis
Do	Analyze the problem, use root cause analysis, and implement solutions
Check	Evaluate solutions
Act	If solutions worked, standardize and implement

SOURCE: Adapted from Sipes, C. (2016). *Project management for the advanced practice nurse.* New York, NY: Springer Publishing Company.

Another component of quality or project control assessment is to continually conduct a review of overall project performance, which means conducting an evaluation of where the project is in terms of how well the project, project team, PM, and all others, including stakeholders, are meeting the project's goals and objectives in a timely, on-budget manner.

Continuous Quality Improvement

There is an increased emphasis on quality in today's healthcare environment, and CQI is something important and essential to any organization but it is particularly important in the healthcare setting. It is essential to examine how things are working to ensure that the best patient care is being provided which can ultimately lead to improvements in patient outcomes (Dearholt & Dang, 2018). Stagnation is never a good thing and it is not good enough to be just satisfied with the status quo. Working toward making improvements should be something that is done on a continual basis.

Quality improvement is a way of reviewing processes and methods to try to continuously make improvement and improve outcomes or quality indicators (Dearholt & Dang, 2018). The methods are reviewed and measured, and then changes are potentially made to improve practice and outcomes, and performance is monitored on an ongoing basis (Dearholt & Dang, 2018). The Affordable Care Act significantly changed the way in which hospitals are reimbursed by linking patient outcomes to the costs for treatment. The Centers for Medicare and Medicaid Services (CMS) now require reporting of quality indicators. Some examples of quality indicators in hospitals are patient falls, hospital-acquired infections (HAIs) such as catheter-associated urinary infections or surgical site infections, patient satisfaction, and hospital readmissions (CMS, 2017). There are definite issues that are inherent in these indicators and speak to the quality of patient care that is being provided.

Today it is common to find healthcare organizations following a new statistical analysis tool and technique known as Six Sigma or Lean methodology. The two of these are often combined and used together in what is known as "Lean Six Sigma." This is a systematic approach that discovers ways to eliminate waste in an organization as well as to improve processes in order to maintain process consistency (Hamilton, 2018). This methodology has its roots in the work of Deming, and these methods are often used in conjunction with the PDCA cycle discussed previously (see Table 6.3).

Deming described systems as interdependent components and processes working together. This description is similar to a healthcare system. Healthcare systems are very complex and adaptive and have many components comprising patients, administrators, and staff (Scoville, Little, Rakover, Luther, & Mate, 2016). Within complex systems, it has been demonstrated that standardizing routine tasks can assist in creating an orderly and stable work environment (Scoville et al., 2016). A stable work environment is needed in order to integrate improvement initiatives and maintain reliable results. One of the most important aspects to CQI and for a stable work environment is for the organization to maintain a culture of change supported by leadership. Healthcare organizations with high-performing management systems are in agreement with Deming that this type of culture is created by and starts with management (Scoville et al., 2016).

The system of healthcare in the United States has changed dramatically over recent years and has shifted from a fee-for-service program to one that is value based with a focus that prevents illnesses, promotes health, and coordinates care (Mason, Gardner, Outlaw, & O'Grady, 2016). This shift requires nurses as well as those in leadership to review the quality indicators mentioned previously in order to look at processes for potential improvement of outcomes. Quality improvement projects in healthcare focus on specific areas of performance, which can lead to improved outcomes as well as waste reduction (Harris, 2018).

Nurses are often at the helm and important strategists in the changes involved in healthcare and quality improvement projects. It is important for the nursing profession to develop its leaders to light the way in regard to change. Part of the strategic plan for healthcare organizations should involve developing new models of care, ensuring nurses have a place at the table in regard to healthcare policy making and advocating for new legislation to improve upon the current laws (Mason et al., 2016).

Dr. Donabedian developed an excellent framework for quality improvement projects in the healthcare setting. The value-based healthcare system that is the focus for today has its roots in Donabedian's framework (Ayanian & Markel, 2016). His framework is based on the triad of structure, processes, and outcomes when evaluating healthcare. The structure piece of the model refers to the qualifications of healthcare professionals or board certifications at an institution and their accrediting agencies. Process or processes are those components by which care is delivered, and outcomes refer to the restoration of function (Ayanian & Markel, 2016).

Key Performance Indicators

You frequently hear about key performance indicators (KPIs), but what is a KPI? A KPI is a business metric—data and numbers used to evaluate factors that are crucial to the success of an organization. When selecting a KPI, it is important to keep it simple with a limited number of KPIs, so that the target can be reached. It also needs to meet the organization's missions and goals. For example, leadership will meet to determine these and invite suggestions from other leaders and managers with the ultimate goal of having three or four KPIs to support the organizational goals and mission. KPIs predict performance and are specifically linked to a strategic objective that helps an organization translate organizational strategy execution into quantifiable terms. When tracking KPIs (data) frequently, changes can be made quickly in order to avoid issues such as moving resources to an area where a task is behind (Chen, n.d.).

Examples of KPIs might be increased patient satisfaction, decreased number of patients left-without-being-seen (LWBS), minutes until patients are seen in the emergency department, and reduced employee turnover by XXX per year if it tracks to the mission statement and goals. Whichever KPIs are selected, they must be measurable and quantifiable and reflect the organization's success. Each KPI must have a target including a due date, the same requirements when developing project objectives.

Metrics

According to Juneja (n.d.), "metrics are numbers that [provide] important information about a process … [and give] accurate measurements about how the process is functioning [to] provide base for … improvements…. Usually measuring results with one metric is not a good enough strategy. A combination of metrics is used to measure the effectiveness of the process" (paras. 1, 3). Metrics can represent anything, but KPIs are said to matter most. KPIs should also be tied to an objective, such as "This will be due on XXX" or "This rate will be reduced by XX%," which is defined by specific objectives that answer the five Ws and an H (Sipes, 2016)—the who, what, where, when, why, and how.

So when is a metric a KPI? KPIs are metrics that meet the five-W criteria. The criteria, the five Ws, should be used in evaluating whether a metric meets KPI status and helps ensure focus on the measures that truly matter to the success of the organization.

In summary, quality control is "a process through which a business seeks to ensure that product quality is maintained or improved with either reduced or zero errors" (Investopedia.com, 2018). The business must establish a working environment where both employees and managers aim for perfection in order to maintain quality control. The main objective of quality control is to ensure that the business is achieving the standards it sets for itself by using tools and processes that provide evidence that supports practice. The method of quality control or management is the process where the quality of completed products is checked for faults by using a number of tools and processes discussed earlier. This usually entails the testing of every product or random samples from each batch if it is not feasible to check every item.

Evidence-Based Practice

The concept of evidence-based practice (EBP) is that it is a combination of the absolute best research combined with patient values along with clinical expertise to produce optimum outcomes (Zimmerman, 2017). EBP often leads to change as nurses look at using the best possible approach to achieve improved quality of care and optimum patient outcomes. As mentioned earlier in this chapter, change can be a difficult process for some. Creating a culture that supports change as well as EBP is essential for the success of an organization in its implementation of quality improvement initiatives. Leadership priorities and resources must align with problems identified by frontline staff (White, 2018). The implementation of EBP by all healthcare providers is extremely important as this does produce safer and more effective care for the patient (Zimmerman, 2017).

Risk Management

As with all monitoring and control processes, all risks must be evaluated for potential negative impact on the overall project. This includes using the many resources available to monitor and track risks including the tools and processes discussed earlier and other tools such as fishbone diagramming, gap analysis, root cause analysis (RCA) processes, and failure mode effect analysis (FMEA) described later in this section. After all tasks have been monitored, assessed, revised, and updated, a report needs to be communicated to all participants in the project including stakeholders and sponsors in a timely manner. A partial list of these tasks is listed here:

- Plan revision—change and update all "living" documents and other project tools. The term "living" document refers to a document that is or may be frequently changed.
- Performance assessment—requires ongoing review of performance from team against the timeline meeting deadlines, against meeting budgets, quality performance with defined metrics in order to track. Question to ask, Is team sacrificing quality to meet deadlines?
- Define and create reports that include status reports previously discussed as well as summary and dashboard reports that provide a quick overview of a topic.

- Utilization of the risk management tool previously defined.

- Monitor scope and change control to provide updated documents and prevent scope creep.

- Control of human resources can be monitored using a tool or tracking document that clearly defines job roles and responsibilities that were identified during the project planning phase. They need to be reviewed, monitored, and controlled during implementations.

- It is important to understand that not all stakeholders should be treated the same––those who have a high impact should be communicated with more frequently and those with low impact can be kept informed.

CASE SCENARIO 6.1

Deb, APRN, PMP, the manager responsible for a very large EHR implementation, has experience with previous implementations but not as large as this one. She is just starting the implementation phase of this project but is uncertain how to monitor for potential risks in such a large project. She begins to discuss this with another more experienced manager. The manager recommends that she review websites and tutorials for risk management tools such as fishbone analysis, SWOT analysis tools and processes, RCA processes and tools, and FMEA processes and tools.

She begins to study and collect the information but still has many questions:

1. How does she apply the tools? Should she assign each of the project team members one of the tasks to start the assessments?

2. What should she do with the information when gathered?

3. Is there some other project where she can observe the actual processes being put in place?

The more experienced manager offers to help guide her through the processes as she implements her project. She will need to document the lessons learned after the implementation is completed (discussed in Chapter 7, Closing the Project—Phase 5).

Another process frequently used when monitoring progress is called "Cause Mapping" or gap analysis (see Figure 6.2). This can be done using an Excel spreadsheet, which is an excellent tool for capturing the elements of a complete root cause analysis (RCA). By changing the way details are documented, a facilitator can improve the entire investigation process. First the problem or gap is identified, a potential cause and effect outlined, and, finally, a solution is explored. There is an excellent healthcare map available free if you currently are using or have Excel on your computers. An example can be found in Figure 6.2.

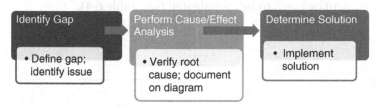

FIGURE 6.2 Cause mapping.
SOURCE: Sipes, C. (2016). *Project management for the advanced practice nurse.* New York, NY: Springer Publishing Company.

Root cause analysis has been mentioned several times. RCA is a "popular and often-used technique to help answer questions of why the problem occurred in the first place. It seeks to identify the origin of a problem using a specific set of steps" (MindTools, 2018) with associated tools such as the fishbone diagram and others, to find the primary cause of the problem, so that you can:

- Establish what happened and why it happened.
- Figure out what to do to reduce the likelihood that it will happen again.

Root cause analysis recognizes that systems and events are interrelated; therefore, an action in one area can lead to and trigger an action in another, and another—creating a domino effect. By tracing back these actions, you can discover where the problem started and how it grew into the issues and problems (MindTools, 2018).

Using the RCA process, issues can be broken down and analyzed further using the fishbone diagram process. The "cause and effect diagram, often called a "fishbone" [(Ishikawa)] diagram, can help in brainstorming to identify possible causes of a problem and in sorting ideas into useful categories. A fishbone diagram is a visual way to look at cause and effect....

[and] is more structured … than some other tools … [that help to identify] causes of a problem" (Medicare, 2018, para. 2).

The problem or effect is displayed at the head or mouth of the fish. Possible contributing causes are sorted on the smaller "bones" under various cause categories (see Figure 6.3). A fishbone diagram can be helpful in identifying possible causes for a problem that might not otherwise be considered an issue by directing the team to look at the categories and think of alternative causes. Next, define and document the real reasons the problem is occurring—what is a symptom of the problem? Include team members who have personal knowledge of the processes and systems involved in the problem or event to be investigated (see Table 6.4).

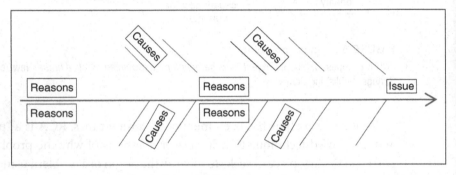

FIGURE 6.3 Root cause analysis: fishbone example.
SOURCE: Sipes, C. (2016). *Project management for the advanced practice nurse.* New York, NY: Springer Publishing Company.

TABLE 6.4 Root Cause Analysis Tracking Tool Using Data From Fishbone

ISSUES AND SOURCE(S)	PROJECTED CAUSE OF ISSUE	SOLUTIONS	RISK IF NOT MITIGATED	ASSIGN OWNER AND DUE DATE
Define the issue and source of cause	What does the group think was the cause based on the investigation?	Recommendations for resolving the problem	High, medium, or low	Who will be responsible for seeing that the issue is resolved?

SOURCE: Sipes, C. (2016). *Project management for the advanced practice nurse.* New York, NY: Springer Publishing Company.

FMEA is a 10-step risk assessment tool and step-by-step process for identifying all possible failures in a design, implementation process, including levels of severity and probability that failure will occur. Examples of the process can be found on the following website: https://sixsigmadsi .com/how-to-complete-the-fmea.

Another important process is the SWOT analysis where the strengths, weaknesses, opportunities, and threats are continually monitored, not only in this phase but also in the implementation and the final closing and evaluation phases. It is important to take advantage of the strengths and opportunities during implementation as well as the continual monitoring of the weaknesses and threats using all of the tools and processes available discussed in this text. Examples of the 10 steps of the SWOT process can be found on the following website: smallbusiness.chron.com/ten -steps-carrying-out-swot-analysis-15451.html.

After the reasons that may have caused the issues have been determined by the project team, the analysis will need to be documented and tracked. Solutions will be recommended, risks assessed if solutions are not implemented, and, finally, critical to the whole process, assignment to an owner with due dates. This can be done by developing a tracking tool in Excel such as the example in Table 6.4.

TESTING

Why Do We Need to Conduct Testing?

As an integral part of quality control, risk management and CQI testing are required to make sure everything that has been built works the way it was designed. There are many, many different types of testing; most cannot be completed before a full system "goes-live." In the case of a very large EHR implementation, random or selected testing is completed. With smaller applications, the entire application can be tested. Whichever level of testing is approved, there must be testing as noted in the many instances of project failure, including the Obama Care failure.

Some of the more common terms associated with testing with which you may be familiar include:

- Unit testing—where the "unit" being developed is tested during the building process
- Integration testing—these are tests completed to make sure the "unit" or application works with other units or applications; that is, it integrates well and does not cause problems

■ System testing—a larger testing process to make sure it not only works with some of the applications but works across the system. For example, do medication orders not only work well within the order placement functionality but flow to all of the areas where an order is needed?

■ Acceptance testing—this type of testing is done by the end users, those who will actually be using the application or system to make sure it meets all expectations

Again there are many types of testing such as load testing where many users are asked to complete a function such as entering orders at the same time to see if the system slows down or even fails during a peak use time. Another type of testing is usability testing where an end user works with the new system to determine how easy it is to use. There are many resources on the web that can provide additional information.

CRITICAL THINKING QUESTIONS AND ACTIVITIES

You need to provide evidence to support some decision-making processes you will implement as you monitor and control implementation of the project you are currently on.

1. What are three of the processes you can use to gather information and data?

2. Which are two of the tools you would use to monitor the project?

You find the tools but do not know how to use them effectively. You also need to demonstrate the use to other team members. Where would you find this information on the Internet? Prepare a presentation for the team based on your findings.

SUMMARY

This chapter on monitoring and controlling the project explained the process and the primary objectives of the process and provided a list of some of the activities that need to be accomplished at the same time as well as ongoing. There was a discussion of how to manage new work that might be discovered as well as a discussion of benefits to monitoring. Most importantly, there was a discussion of why projects fail. By understanding what lessons and reasons for failure have been found in other projects, it should help to manage expectations with the current project. Quality control methods and CQI were discussed with examples of tools that can be used to monitor quality or suggestions for creating your own tools, listing the key elements that need to be controlled. Finally, a summary of why testing is critically needed was provided, including a discussion of some of the most common terms.

REFERENCES

Arveson, P. (1998). *The Deming cycle.* Retrieved from https://balancedscorecard.org/Resources/Articles-White-Papers/The-Deming-Cycle

Ayanian, J. Z., & Markel, H. (2016). Donabedian's lasting framework for health care quality. *New England Journal of Medicine, 375*(3), 205–207. doi:10.1056/NEJMp1605101

Carlos, T. (2018). *Reasons why projects fail.* Retrieved from https://www.projectsmart.co.uk/reasons-why-projects-fail.php

Centers for Medicare & Medicaid Services. (2017). *Hospital quality initiative: Outcome measures.* Retrieved from https://www.cms.gov/Medicare/Quality-Initiatives-Patient-Assessment-Instruments/HospitalQualityInits/OutcomeMeasures.html

Chen, N. (n.d.). *KPIs are more than just metrics* [Blog post]. Retrieved from https://www.repsly.com/blog/consumer-goods/kpis-are-more-than-just-metrics

Dearholt, S., & Dang, D. (2018). *Johns Hopkins nursing evidence based practice: Model and guidelines* (3rd ed.). Indianapolis, IN: Sigma Theta Tau International.

Hamilton, L. (2018, January 25). Lean, lean six sigma and the clinical laboratory. *Medical Laboratory Observer,* 42–43. Retrieved from https://www.mlo-online.com/lean-lean-six-sigma-clinical-laboratory

Harris, A. M. (2018, July 20). Field report: Mapping a start for quality improvement. *Physician Leadership Journal.* Retrieved from https://www.physicianleaders.org/news/field-report-mapping-a-start-for-quality-improvement

Investopedia.com. (2018). *Quality control.* Retrieved from https://www.investopedia.com

Juneja, P. (n.d.). What are metrics and why are they important? ManagementStudyGuide.com. Retrieved from https://www.managementstudyguide.com/what-are-metrics.htm

Mason, D., Gardner, D., Hopkins Outlaw, F., & O'Grady, E. (Eds.). (2016). *Policy & politics in nursing and healthcare* (7th ed.). St. Louis, MO: Elsevier.

Medicare. (2018). *How to use the fishbone tool for root cause analysis.* Retrieved from https://www.cms.gov/medicare/provider-enrollment-and-certification/qapi/downloads/fishbonerevised.pdf

MindTools. (2018). *Root cause analysis: Tracing a problem to its origins.* Retrieved from https://www.mindtools.com/pages/article/newTMC_80.htm

Reh, J. (2018). *Pareto's principle or the 80/20 rule.* Retrieved from https://www.thebalancecareers.com/pareto-s-principle-the-80-20-rule-2275148

Scoville, R., Little, K., Rakover, J., Luther, K., & Mate, K. (2016). *Sustaining improvement* [IHI White Paper]. Cambridge, MA: Institute for Healthcare Improvement.

Retrieved from http://www.ihi.org/resources/Pages/IHIWhitePapers/Sustaining-Improvement.aspx

Sipes, C. (2016). *Project management for the advanced practice nurse*. New York, NY: Springer Publishing Company.

White, K. (2018). What is transformational leadership? A model for sparking innovation. *CIO*. Retrieved from https://www.cio.com/article/3257184/what-is-transformational-leadership-a-model-for-motivating-innovation.html

Zimmerman, K. (2017). Essentials of evidence based practice. *International Journal of Childbirth Education*, 32(2), 37–43.

CHAPTER 7

CLOSING THE PROJECT— PHASE 5

Upon completion of this chapter, the reader will be able to:

1. Define three processes of the closing phase.
2. Discuss types of project closure.
3. Discuss three tasks to be accomplished during the closing phase.
4. Discuss the purpose of the project close-out meeting.
5. Discuss the value of analyzing lessons learned at the close of the project.
6. Discuss when the closing functions should be implemented.
7. Discuss the value of the final report, who is responsible, and who receives it.

- Key Terms
- Introduction
- Closing Phases of a Project
- Closing Tasks to Complete
- Project Close-Out Meeting

- Formal Acceptance
- Final Report
- Summary

KEY TERMS

- Closing
- Debrief
- Lessons learned
- Review of deliverables
- Transition
- Verification audit

INTRODUCTION

Closing can be a conflict between the very busy times on the project and moving on to something different, even another project. Whether it is an internal or external project, you must have met the constraints discussed in earlier chapters that were defined for the project. If it is an internal project closing, you must seamlessly transition the project into the company's normal operations. For external projects such as a small project (wedding) or larger project (work related), check formal documents to make sure all deadlines and budgets have been met. Final delivery of the product should be reviewed to make sure it meets the needs and expectations of the organization (Closing Process Groups, 2012; Aziz, 2015).

During the closing phase, the tasks that need to be completed include debriefing the team, transitioning all of the appropriate documentation and project history, as well as transitioning all activities back to those who will own, support, and maintain the activity. The primary objective of the closing and transition processes is to obtain formal acceptance of the completed project by the project champion and key stakeholders if indicated. The transition and closing documents are discussed more in detail with examples later in this chapter (Closing Process Group, 2018, p. 1).

> ▶ QUESTIONS TO CONSIDER BEFORE
>   READING ON
> ■ What are some reasons for project closure?
> ■ What are types/reasons for project closure?
> ■ Discuss the steps to closing the project.
> ■ What are some potential problems if the project is
>   not closed properly?

CLOSING PHASES OF A PROJECT

There are several steps to the closing process. One of the processes is closing the project *phase*, which can be one of two steps—completing and closing the *full project* or *termination* of the project that may not have been fully competed due to some reasons, such as lack of funding, leadership support, or many other reasons.

It is also important to understand why it is essential to close the project in a formal way, as there could be liability issues if not done properly regardless of the size of the project. Following is a list of other reasons a project can be closed, but regardless of the reason for the closure, critical questions need to be addressed (see Table 7.1).

TABLE 7.1 Types of Project Closure

TYPES OF PROJECT CLOSURE	CLOSE-OUT PLAN: QUESTIONS TO ASK
■ Normal ■ Premature ■ Perpetual ■ Failed project ■ Changed priority	■ What tasks are required to close the project? ■ Who will be responsible for these tasks? ■ When will closure begin and end? ■ How will the project be delivered?

SOURCE: Sipes, C. (2019). *Project management for the advanced practice nurse* (2nd ed.). New York, NY: Springer Publishing Company.

Even if a project is put on hold, terminated early, or even considered a failure, the project manager (PM) is still responsible for properly closing the project and making sure all tasks are completed or assigned to a different owner who will be responsible for follow-up.

According to *A Guide to the Project Management Body of Knowledge (PMBOK Guide)*, "the Project Closing Process Group consists of processes performed to conclude all activities across all ... [g]roups to formally complete the project, phase, or contractual obligations. [The Closing] Process Group, when completed, verifies that the defined processes are completed within all of the Process Groups to close the project or a project phase, as appropriate, and formally establishes that the project or project phase is complete" (Closing Process Group—Project Management Resources, 2018, p. 1; Aziz, 2015; see Figure 7.1).

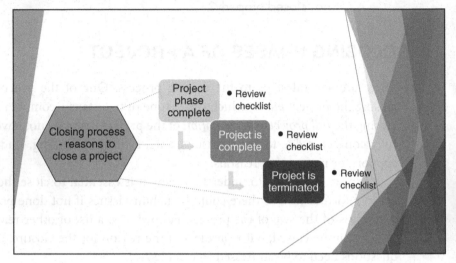

FIGURE 7.1 Project management process: steps in closing process.
SOURCE: Sipes, C. (2019). *Project management for the advanced practice nurse* (2nd ed.). New York, NY: Springer Publishing Company.

You may be wondering why it is important to close a project following legal recommendations—some of the issues were discussed earlier.

- Frequently, most PMs organize project closing at the end of a project, some many times during the life of a project, and others never at all. But what is the liability to the organization when a project is not closed properly or even not at all? The PM must understand the consequences if the project is not closed properly.

Project closing *must definitely* occur at the *end of the project*. This also includes termination since this will be the end of the project. However, the best practice is that closing needs to occur at *every phase* in the project life cycle, which is the process you started in your first practicum where you developed the Kick-Off presentation at the conclusion of the *planning phase* and then last term as you evaluated and documented milestones met as you began to close the *implementation phase*. Phase definition may be logical, preferential, or even hypothetical. When devising project phases, three factors need to be taken into consideration:

■ What can happen if the project is not properly closed? If not properly closed, it can leave the organization liable to external parties for incomplete payments on contracts, and liable to customers/stakeholders for not meeting the legal scope requirements signed off by leadership.

There are a number of steps that must be followed in an organized way to make sure all areas of the project have been addressed and there are no gaps in the processes. This includes asking questions and documentation of findings. See Box 7.1 for a partial list of key areas and questions that need to be assessed and addressed during project closure. The list depends on the organization and size of the project and organizational requirements.

BOX 7.1

QUESTIONS AND STEPS REQUIRED DURING FINAL CLOSURE PROCESS

Project Closure: Types of Closure

Steps:

■ Have you made sure all of the work needed and contracted been completed?

■ Is approval by the project's sponsor and customer—internal or external—complete?

■ Have all organizational governance processes been executed?

■ Have defined/expected project management processes been applied?

■ Has administrative closing of all procurements and contracts been completed by both parties; have all contractual obligations toward each other been completed/signed off?

■ Has completion of project been formally recognized including transition of operations?

■ Have benefits of project been validated against the business case?

■ Have Lessons Learned been completed, including what could have been done better, documented, and reported to leadership?

■ Have project resources been disbanded, freeing them for other projects?

■ Have all project deliverables to the customer been transitioned demonstrating seamless operations and support?

SOURCE: Sipes, C. (2019). *Project management for the advanced practice nurse* (2nd ed.). New York, NY: Springer Publishing Company.

Additional questions might include:

- Have all lessons learned from each closing phase been documented, including planning, implementation, monitor, and control phases?
- Did all stakeholders have an opportunity to provide input and feedback including end users?
- Was a final review by all owners and stakeholders of all original, legal documents, and requirements conducted to determine success of meeting these critical success factors (CSFs) and milestones?
- Has an area, archive, library for storage of all project documents, accessible to all stakeholders, been established?

Finally, the last steps of closing a project—those of Project Completion and Project Termination—require final assessments of the project status such as any outstanding tasks that need to be completed, feedback from stakeholders, paying vendors, closing final contracts, and other tasks.

▶ **QUESTIONS TO CONSIDER BEFORE READING ON**

1. What does a verification audit entail?
2. Why do you need to complete a verification audit?
3. What are some other closing tasks that must be completed?

CLOSING TASKS TO COMPLETE

Verification Audit

This audit is a report that summarizes that the products purchased at the beginning of the project were received and working correctly. In addition, these audits should have been conducted throughout the controlling phase of the project. Anything unexpected or out of scope will need to be discussed with leadership and approved with sign-off during this audit.

Sign-Off With Leadership

The final sign-off with leadership validates that there is agreement with the products purchased, the functionality and user acceptance testing (UAT), change requests approved, and all other items listed in the scope document.

The report is also shared with all leadership and sponsors and any other businesses involved in the project to provide input and verify that all tasks and outcomes of the project were met (Table 7.2).

TABLE 7.2 Verification Audit Document

VERIFICATION AUDIT TASK/PRODUCT	OWNER	SIGNATURE/ SPONSOR/DATE
Products (purchased list)		

Functionality/user acceptance testing
  – Can product be used/function as designed?
  – Does it meet business needs?		

Change requests approved		
Other tasks from scope document		
Does final project meet success measures outlined in scope document?		
Were all requirements outlined in project plan met?		

SOURCE: Sipes, C. (2016). *Project management for the advanced practice nurse.* New York, NY: Springer Publishing Company.

Review of Final Deliverables

The PM must review responses and determine if final sign-off is acceptable. If not, then a meeting needs to be scheduled with all involved—leadership, sponsors, and end users—to determine how best to resolve all and any issues to make it acceptable. It should include review of documents, including documents on risk, change, budget, constraints, and assumptions. Specifically, the budget needs to be checked with the key person responsible for the overall budget, including each line item reviewed against original estimates; after this has been completed satisfactorily, the budget must be signed off.

All documents listed in the scope and charter documents must be reviewed and discussed with key stakeholders and sponsors to make sure all tasks and processes have been reviewed and completed. Other key documents that need to be reviewed and signed off during this meeting include the work breakdown structure (WBS) and Gantt chart.

Lessons Learned

What Are Lessons Learned? "Lessons learned" is a term frequently used by anyone completing a project—it is a time to review, collect, and document information regarding how things went and what can be improved for the next project as well as getting feedback from everyone involved in the project. This is set up as a meeting where it is expected that everyone will be in attendance and contribute to the final assessment. Things that need to be improved upon will be documented and assigned an owner in case there is a need for further resolution.

The outcome of this meeting is to prepare a final report for leadership and stakeholders. The lessons-learned session is usually set up in a meeting or conference room. All who have been involved in the project will be invited to provide comment. One way to do this is to go around the table and have everyone share his or her insights while minutes are being recorded.

Another more confidential and productive way to collect information is to send out meeting invitations to those who wish to be included in the evaluation process and have them come to an open room where large sheets of paper are put up around the room. The large Post-its will have various topics listed at the top. Then attendees write comments on sticky notes and place them under the topic of choice.

After everyone has had a chance to provide input, collect and tabulate the data and prepare the report. Other objectives of the lessons-learned function are to:

- Define additional work that needs to be done
- Determine if there are other changes that need to be made to the project, its processes, or methodology
- Define customer satisfaction with the deliverable and value and benefits of the project
- Review the quality and performance of the project and teams (see Box 7.2)

BOX 7.2

LESSONS-LEARNED PROCESS EXAMPLE

- **Topic:** Functionality of clinical documentation
    - It was great!
    - It did not function as advertised—it did not do XXXXX
    - It would be better if …
    - XXX is missing

(continued)

- **Topic:** Med order process
  - Med ordering did not show correct times
  - Too many clicks to get to the area to enter orders
  - Sign-off function did not work well

SOURCE: Sipes, C. (2016). *Project management for the advanced practice nurse.* New York, NY: Springer Publishing Company.

Transition of Project Documents and Plans: Transition Plans

Why do you need a transition plan or handoff? Project transition is also referred to as "knowledge transfer" because it involves educating the new owners of the project tasks on the key elements of the project: what went well, and what might need further work or revisions. Closing a project includes a number of activities and tasks that need to be completed by the PM as well as the project team. A number of the project closing documents will have been completed as discussed earlier; now it is time to review to make sure everything has been completed and a plan is in place for archiving the documents as well as the formal handoff to the new owners of tasks that might need to be completed yet or maintained. In addition to developing the project closing documents, which will include the milestones and verification audit, you will also need to develop a transition and hand-off plan.

The transition plan is important in that it will provide the stakeholders, leadership, and team members with information on the project completion and transition back to anyone who might continue with other phases or optimization of the same project. The final documents should be kept in a file where all management documents are kept. Information and documents included in the transition plan will describe the transfer of any outstanding work that remains that will be completed in the next phase or goes to information technology support or a designee to oversee any maintenance that might be needed.

The final meeting should be set up and include the project sponsor and stakeholders, if appropriate, and others from the project team. Tasks include preparing an agenda including the intent of a meeting to review the lists of all documents that will be turned over to the new owners, and key highlights of what transpired during the four or five different phases of the project. It is also important to emphasize the turnover and hand-off to the new owners who will formally sign off at the conclusion of the meeting, which indicates they understand the project has ended from your perspective.

The transition documents should include:

- Final report
- A list of all presentations related to the project
- A list of files, documents, and reports
- A list of all deliverables including documentation of processes and change reports
- Maintenance and system requirements going forward
- Identification of any additional work that needs to be completed as well as all documents that have been completed, including status reports, risk management plans, and other documented tasks; create an "open issues and incomplete tasks" report

These documents should be prepared in both paper and electronic formats. The project sponsors will indicate where they want the documents archived (Project Closure, n.d., pp. 1–3).

Final Analysis and Debriefing

The final analysis and debriefing is an important step—overlooked by many as too time consuming. But this process provides an opportunity to review the project's successes and failures. It also provides opportunities to add success measures that are not already defined. During this meeting, it will be important to review the outcome and value of the project, review additional work if needed, review deficiencies, recommend changes for processes that did not work, and review the quality of the project and overall satisfaction of the project.

▶ **QUESTIONS TO CONSIDER BEFORE READING ON**

- What are additional tasks required to close a project?
- What is the purpose of the project close-out meeting?

PROJECT CLOSE-OUT MEETING

In project termination, one of the final tasks to be completed is the checklist for the project close-out meeting. The purpose of this meeting is to make sure there is a seamless transfer of knowledge to the identified new owner. It is important to review all steps from the scope, charter, and other documents as well as discuss lessons learned collected and documented at end of each phase of the project (Landau, 2017). All project deliverables will need to be reviewed and documented on the verification audit form discussed below before final, official, legal acceptance, and then with sign-off of key stakeholders and sponsors, the project can be closed (see Box 7.3).

BOX 7.3

PROJECT CLOSE-OUT MEETING TASKS CHECKLIST

- What is the purpose and objectives of the final meeting?
- What tasks need to be completed before the meeting?
- Who should attend the meeting? List attendees.
- What tasks need to be completed during the meeting such as owner assignments?
- What tasks need follow-up after the meeting?
- What are the next steps?

SOURCE: Sipes, C. (2019). *Project management for the advanced practice nurse* (2nd ed.). New York, NY: Springer Publishing Company.

The objective of the checklist for the project close-out meeting is to review and document all activities creating a final project close-out report at the end of the meetings with all stakeholders and sponsors in attendance. The report will contain documentation of any potential outstanding activities and tasks that are assigned to the right people, including who the owners are, and should capture the 5Ws and an H (Sipes, 2016), including:

- What went well?
- Did the project meet all the constraints including on time, on budget, and quality?
- Did the lessons-learned process include recommendations for future actions to create success?

- What and how were challenges met; what can be done better?
- How were risks managed; what could be done better?
- Were roles and responsibilities clear?
- How can knowledge and experiences learned here best be transferred to other projects and teams?
- What recommendations should be shared with other PMs and teams?

Tasks that need to be completed before the meeting should have been outlined during the planning phase, even as an anticipated overview of the project. The meeting should occur right after deliverables have been completed and should be identified as part of the project deliverables—always planning ahead.

The meeting date should be set in agreement with the main attendees' schedules and include the project team and manager, project sponsor, and key stakeholders. Be sure there is a structured meeting procedure, including an agenda, and review this at the beginning of the meeting. Everyone should have received the agenda in advance, which includes:

- Purpose of meeting
- Introduction of all attendees
- Overview of the project
- High-level evaluation of project, value/impact, and feedback
- Discussion of lessons learned
- Next steps inducing new owners
- Official project closure including sign-off of formal documents and verification audit

A final activity of project termination will need an agenda sent out to all attendees prior to the final official closing including a short slide presentation (8–10 slides) to keep the meeting organized. In the presentation, show relevant documents completed during implementation of the project, such as the project plan, scope, requirements documents such as the risk management tool and responsible, accountable, consulted, informed (RACI) chart, data analysis, and project close-out checklist (Table 7.3), which have been prepared in advance and will be discussed in the meeting.

One of the slides should include the project milestone status checklist the team has prepared to discuss. It includes the project milestones' status—success and areas for improvement, which provides a quick review of overall project status at close-out (see Table 7.3).

TABLE 7.3 Project Milestone Status Checklist

DESCRIPTION OF TASK	STATUS	OWNER	DATE COMPLETED	NOTES
Outstanding issues documented/resolved	At risk			
All tasks identified in WBS completed	Completed			
Goals met	Overdue			
End users trained	On hold			
Measures of success measured and communicated	Overdue			
Feedback from stakeholders documented and communicated	Completed			
Project team evaluated and released	Overdue			

WBS, work breakdown structure.

SOURCE: Sipes, C. (2019). *Project management for the advanced practice nurse* (2nd ed.). New York, NY: Springer Publishing Company.

As discussed earlier, allow time for discussion of areas for improvement and recommendations from lessons learned to be applied to future projects. Encourage discussion of what went wrong, how it can be improved, for example, by changing a process, methods, or resources. Postmeeting write-up should include minutes of decisions and action items/next steps as well as owners. Once the minutes have been approved and sent out to all attendees, a follow-up with a close-out report that the PM develops is sent to all stakeholders including the project team and the report is added to the final project folder and ready to be filed where all future teams can access it.

- Discuss next steps:
  - Outstanding tasks or project follow-up activities
  - Creating final close-out report
  - Making project documentation, including close-out report, available to future projects and teams, that is, retain knowledge

After officially closing the project, mark project as "finished" with official sign-off and be sure to acknowledge team's and individual achievements. Then finally, celebrate the team and project success.

In summary, the final steps of closing a project—those of project completion and project termination—require final assessments of the project status such as any outstanding tasks that need to be completed, feedback from stakeholders, paying vendors, closing final contracts, and other tasks as discussed earlier, using the tools developed during the different phases of the project.

It will be interesting to review the information collected as the report is prepared. An important process during lessons learned is to have all project team members involved in preparing the final report so they can review the comments.

When all documentation is completed, a final report will be prepared for leadership and stakeholders. A summary of tasks completed and outcomes of the project includes preparation of the documents including the final report, delivery of all working documents, preparation of the final presentation, and a documented transition plan with formal handoff and knowledge transfer with owners identified. A review of the CSFs for the project and outcome of the meeting will need to be documented as well (Linky, 2010).

> ► **QUESTIONS TO CONSIDER BEFORE READING ON**
> 1. What is formal acceptance?
> 2. How is the formal acceptance used to create the final report?

FORMAL ACCEPTANCE

What is "formal acceptance"? Not only is preparing all final documents during the closing phase an important task but also getting formal and final sign-off from the project sponsors is a must. When this process is complete, it indicates the sponsors have reviewed all of the documentation provided, have discussed and understood the issues and recommendations presented, and now accept the final report with a signature (Table 7.4).

TABLE 7.4 Project Modifications During Project Implementation

ORIGINAL MILE-STONES FROM SCOPE	MODIFICATION STATUS	FINAL MILESTONES
		Agreement:
		Sign-off date:

SOURCE: Sipes, C. (2016). *Project management for the advanced practice nurse.* New York, NY: Springer Publishing Company.

The report should include a review of the key milestones from the original scope and charter documents, the due dates for those, and whether they were adjusted and how they were met. If there were revisions of the milestones, those will need to be included in the report (see Table 7.5). It will be critical to obtain a signature to verify the review of the documents and activities, and formally conclude the meeting.

CASE SCENARIO 7.1

In the final closing phases of the project, Jon has completed most of the closing activities including collecting all of the reports and reviewing all of the data and information in the project management tools. He had just completed the project close-out meeting but there were a number of follow-up items that needed to be completed.

Jon is not sure how to complete the rest of the deliverables and now asks the senior leadership what his next steps should be.

The CEO directs Jon to set up another meeting with just leadership and legal advisors to make sure there is final documentation of all that occurred in the meeting and the next steps that were outlined in the meeting. Remaining questions with which Jon will need assistance include:

- Where will the resources come from to help finalize last steps?
- What is the new timeline now for the final small tasks needed for final legal sign-off by both the organization and vendors?

FINAL REPORT

The final report should provide details about the project and members of the organization who were involved in the project, if applicable. The report should be prepared as a document with consideration that the persons reading it may not be familiar with the project. They should be able to read the report and know the "who" involved and at what level, what was done, how it was done, and why the project was needed (Rowley, 2018).

The content will need to be clear, concise, and consistent and contain meaningful information that aligns with the scope documents. If the organization has a standard format for documentation, that must be used. One goal for the report is to include notation that there were tangible deliverables that were clear, insightful, on time, and within budget that were outlined in the project charter.

The basic outline for the document should follow the project life cycle in terms of what happened in each phase of the project and focus on:

- Background of needs
- Project expectations that were consistent with scope
- List of deliverables defined in the project charter
- Preparation of the final report that includes past reports
- Review of potential content of the final report with a project steering team, or other key stakeholder who has been supportive of the project, if there is one.

An example of the final report document is provided in Table 7.5.

TABLE 7.5 Final Report Document

FINAL REPORT—DATE OF REPORT	PROJECT MANAGER (INCLUDE WHO PREPARED THE REPORT IF DESIGNATED)
Title Page: (Client name, location, project title)	
Table of Contents	
Executive Summary: (Organization, purpose, project objective, main outcomes, key recommendations)	
Background and Objectives: (Organization, project objectives, reason for project, issues and documented need, expected results)	

(continued)

TABLE 7.5 Final Report Document (*continued*)

FINAL REPORT—DATE OF REPORT	PROJECT MANAGER (INCLUDE WHO PREPARED THE REPORT IF DESIGNATED)
Approach: (Detail scope of project, implementation process with tasks—can include WBS as appendix and refer to it)	
Findings: (Summary of findings—refer to WBS—add other appendices with references to them)	
Recommendations: (Based on key findings and issues)	
Conclusion: (Summarize/discuss approach and processes used, project objectives, issues with resolutions)	
Appendices	

WBS, work breakdown structure.

SOURCE: Sipes, C. (2016). *Project management for the advanced practice nurse.* New York, NY: Springer Publishing Company.

The final report will be presented as one formal, professional document with all additional documents added as appendices and noted in the table of contents. It will be important to include all documents bound together as one or in a notebook. It is difficult, appears disorganized, and is more time consuming if there are many separate documents to review.

CRITICAL THINKING QUESTIONS AND ACTIVITIES

Discuss the project termination steps and strategies.

- Why is it important to have a formal project closing and termination?

Search the website to find documents that you would need to complete the formal close-out of a project.

- Other than the documents provided in the text, what other forms and documents will you need?

If you have had experiences with an electronic health record (EHR) project implementation, describe your current experiences so far with closing the final phase of the project: issues, challenges, and successes with support from the scholarly literature.

SUMMARY

The closing phase of the project indicates the different tasks of the project that have been completed and now ready for handoff and transition to the original organization or party, whoever originally requested the project. This chapter introduced the final processes necessary to formally and legally close out a project and included the description of the verification audit with an example of a verification audit tool. It also provided a discussion of project deliverables, lessons-learned processes, and a lessons-learned tool to use during the final meeting.

A description of elements needed in the final report as well as the final report tool was provided, along with the discussion of what should be included in the transition plan and transition documents. The final three topics include the final analysis and debriefing, formal acceptance, and a project modification during the project. A PM will use any or all of these tools. Many of the tools were developed, altered, and revised for use on many different and varied projects, both large and small, from very large to much smaller organizations and health systems.

REFERENCES

Aziz, E. E. (2015). *Project closing: The small process group with big impact.* Paper presented at PMI® Global Congress 2015—EMEA, London, England. Newtown Square, PA: Project Management Institute.

Closing Process Group—Bright Hub Project Management. (2018). Retrieved from http://www.brighthubpm.com

Closing Process Group—Project Management Resources. (2018). Retrieved from http://www.villanovau.com/resources/project-management/pmbok-closing-process-group/#.VdYeOLJViko (p. 1).

Closing Process Groups. (2012). Retrieved from http://www.villanovau.com/resources/project-management/pmbok-closing-process-group/#.VdYeOLJViko

Landau, P. (2017). The *ultimate project closure checklist* [Blog post]. Retrieved from https://www.projectmanager.com/blog/project-closure-checklist

Linky. (2010). *Project management closure: Best practice for project learning.* Retrieved from http://www.virtualprojectconsulting.com/project-management-closure-best-practice

Project closure—Whether your 1st or 21st project, successful completion involves a few important steps.... (n.d.). Retrieved from http://www.mastering-project-management.com/project-closure.html

Rowley, J. (2018). *PMBOK® Guide–Process 4.7 Close Project or Phase: Inputs* (6th ed.). Retrieved from https://4squareviews.com/2018/02/15/6th-edition-pmbok-guide-process

Sipes, C. (2016). *Project management for the advanced practice nurse.* New York, NY: Springer Publishing Company.

Sipes, C. (2019). *Project management for the advanced practice nurse* (2nd ed.). New York, NY: Springer Publishing Company.

SECTION III

APPLICATION OF PROJECT MANAGEMENT CONCEPTS AND TOOLS

CHAPTER 8

CASE STUDIES: APPLYING PROJECT MANAGEMENT CONCEPTS AND TOOLS

TONI HEBDA | CAROLYN SIPES

LEARNING OBJECTIVES

Upon completion of this chapter, the reader will be able to:

1. Discuss two project management tasks a nurse practitioner (NP) would need in practice.

2. List three project management skills a chief nursing informatics officer (CNIO) would use.

3. Differentiate between project management skills needed by a nurse executive (NE) versus a nurse manager.

4. Discuss the project management tools and processes a clinical nurse specialist (CNS) might use to start up a new clinic.

5. Describe three of the nine steps a doctor of nursing practice (DNP) will take to develop a project in the doctorate program that is required for graduation.

6. Describe one exemplar where the success of a coordinator of a high-fidelity simulation lab might be enhanced through the use of project management to set up and manage a high-fidelity skills lab.

7. Provide examples of how the use of project management by a nurse educator could facilitate the design, management, and evaluation of simulations for use across a degree program.

8. Discuss project management knowledge and skills that a provider such as a DNP and other advanced practice registered nurses (APRNs) might employ to select a new office electronic health record.

OUTLINE

- Key Terms
- Introduction
- How the APRN, DNP, Nurse Educator, and Other Healthcare Professional Roles With Advanced Preparation Would Use Project Management Concepts
- Summary

KEY TERMS

- Advanced practice registered nurse (APRN)
- Chief nursing informatics officer (CNIO)
- Chief nursing officer (CNO)
- Clinical nursing specialist (CNS)
- Doctor of nursing practice (DNP)
- Informatics nurse specialist (INS)
- Nurse educator
- Nurse executive (NE)
- Nurse practitioner (NP)
- Other healthcare professionals

INTRODUCTION

The majority of nursing students will tell you that they have never had a class in project management nor have they had an opportunity to lead a project, unless they have had occasion to implement technology in a practicum setting. However, there are expectations today for all nurses, particularly those with advanced levels of education, to practice to the fullest extent allowed by their individual scopes of practice. Working at these levels allows nurses to fill gaps in practice and lead a variety of initiatives geared to improve coordination of care, outcomes, and workflow. The ability to plan, lead, and later evaluate these initiatives is enhanced through familiarity with project management techniques. The nursing process provides an ideal foundation for project management techniques.

Frequent comments heard are that project management is not taught in nursing school because it is something required in business. However, the nursing process provides an ideal foundation for project management techniques. The nursing process is a systematic method of assessment, diagnosis, planning, implementation, and evaluation. Project management is very similar and encompasses comparable procedures and processes. Although nurses may not receive formal training on business topics, there are many skills they do learn that can help them conceive and manage projects in the workplace.

There are many roles that the APRN educator and other healthcare professionals with advanced preparation can assume, given the opportunity to develop knowledge and skills needed for a particular role or job (Bovero, Giacomo, Ansari, & Roulin, 2018). APRNs can meet challenges presented by evolving healthcare.

The intent of this chapter is to suggest and demonstrate by example how different tasks associated with the different roles the APRN, DNPs, as well as other nurses and healthcare professionals with advanced education can assume and apply in practice (Association of College & Research Libraries, 2015). There is a belief that nurses and other healthcare professionals do not or will not use project management concepts in practice; however, there are many terms that are consistent in both project management and nursing practice, such as the nursing process. The different case studies presented here will add clarity to project management terms when the overlap in semantics is noted.

Literature suggests that APRNs, DNPs, and other practitioners in advanced practice roles today are not adequately or uniformly prepared for advanced leadership roles, despite expectations that they will lead healthcare reform and initiatives to improve care (Culbertson & Jackson, 2016; Delgado & Mitchell, 2016; Eliades, Jakubik, Weese, & Huth, 2017; Holle & Kornusky, 2018; Reichard & Walker, 2016). This lack of readiness to lead can be attributed to a variety of factors that include, but are not limited to, a lack of qualified faculty, a lack of motivation and readiness for leadership development, whether the individual sees oneself as a leader, the level of support provided for leadership development, opportunities to actively practice leadership skills, and curriculum gaps (Aarons, Ehrhart, Farahnak, & Hurlburt, 2015). A lack of readiness to lead can negatively impact work preparation satisfaction, lead to higher rates of turnover, and disrupt the environment (Kenny, Reeve, & Hall, 2016).

One of the skills identified in the literature for leaders is informatics competencies (Kennedy & Moen, 2017; Kleib, Simpson, & Rhodes, 2016), yet deficits remain in informatics knowledge among faculty and in the curricula leaving graduates with insufficient knowledge of information technology (IT) to lead effective design and use to support decisions (Collins, Yen, Phillips, & Kennedy, 2017; Oakes, Frisch, Potter, & Borycki, 2015). This situation has forced leaders to gain the informatics knowledge and skills needed through on-the-job learning and various professional development activities. Project management is a foundational concept in informatics, although the skills that come under this umbrella today have been used by nurses in a variety of ways for a number of years. For example, having the ability to log on and document in a computer where the computer is the primary mode of entering patient data has been a function nurses have assumed for a number of years. Historically, nursing education did not include informatics competencies; thus, current managers, administrators, or nurse executives (NEs) may not be adequately prepared to use or lead change in the use of health information technology (HIT; Westra & Delaney, 2008).

HOW THE APRN, DNP, NURSE EDUCATOR, AND OTHER HEALTHCARE PROFESSIONAL ROLES WITH ADVANCED PREPARATION WOULD USE PROJECT MANAGEMENT CONCEPTS

Holle and Kornusky (2018) noted that leadership is critical to achieve quality care. One way to achieve quality care is through the ability to lead others through the implementation of innovation (Aarons et al., 2015).

National nursing organizations' leadership have taken steps to define skills needed in many nursing roles; some examples of APRN roles and application of skills that will be needed can be found here. One such example is from the American Organization of Nurse Executives (AONE, 2015). AONE calls for skills in communication and business, all of which overlap with leadership competencies. The AONE's Nursing Executive Competencies lists skills in communication and business skills, all of which overlap with leadership competencies. AONE has dedicated a section to information management and technology under business skills to improve performance, inform decisions, evaluate data quality, recognize trends applicable to patient care, and lead adoption of technology and later evaluate its success. Another national organization, Healthcare Information and Management Systems Society (HIMSS, 2013), states that, "Nursing leaders must have computer and informatics knowledge and skills to work with other disciplines" and previously had an NE workgroup and a toolkit for that population to develop informatics competencies (Pope, 2016). That workgroup no longer exists but there is an HIMSS Project Management special interest group that exists to "provide opportunities for collaboration and professional development of project managers in healthcare organizations" which it supports through networking, education, and a variety of resources (HIMSS, 2018, para. 1).

APRN, DNP, and Other Healthcare Professional Roles: Where Concepts Apply

There are 11 examples and case studies of different roles where an APRN, DNP, and other nurses and healthcare professionals with advanced educational preparation will need to utilize project management concepts and tools in his or her practice. The roles include the nurse administrator as an NE or nurse manager, a nurse practitioner (NP), a clinical nursing specialist (CNS), an informatics nurse specialist (INS), a chief nursing informatics officer (CNIO), a chief nursing officer (CNO), and a doctor of nursing practice (DNP) student in the final practicum before graduation, a simulation center coordinator, nurse educator, and a provider.

Case Studies: Nurse Administrator

NE

Becky R. has an MSN and is the new NE for ABC Medical Center, a 35-bed, medical–surgical department. She is in charge of 55 RNs and patient care technicians (PCTs). Becky was just recently promoted from the nurse manager position to the NE position. In this position, she brings a number of skills she acquired as the nurse manager but also is expected to have additional leadership skills including:

- Manage finances—cost containment
- Provide oversight for operational and capital budgets
- Determine cost–benefit analysis and unit budget control measures
- Understand financial resource procurement and develop monitoring plans
- Develop and set measureable objectives
- Identify key stakeholders for projects
- Prepare reports, metrics, tables, graphs/charts, and dashboard reports
- Propose actions, build on past lessons learned
- Monitor outcomes
- Develop and understand workflow processes
- Manage time
- Be consistent; have consistent processes
- Provide and understand organizational governance
- Monitor quality improvement

In Becky's previous job as the nurse manager, she had the opportunity to take two PM courses at the university where she became more proficient in such skills as developing communication plans, communicating with organizational leadership through report writing, and attending meetings where she also learned to work well with group process. She learned to develop change management plans and by doing so utilized the change process to become more knowledgeable in team building and managing conflict, while providing resolutions and managing resources; she became more computer literate as well. All of the skills she developed aided in her promotion to NE (Chapter 3, Design/Initiation: Project Management—Phase 1, and Chapter 4, Planning: Project Management—Phase 2).

One of the conditions for her promotion was that she would need to take further courses to learn how to manage finances—cost containment, provide oversight for operational and capital budgets, determine cost–benefit analysis and unit budget control measures, understand financial resource procurement, and develop monitoring plans that also include monitoring quality improvement (Chapter 4, Planning: Project Management—Phase 2, to Chapter 6, Monitoring and Controlling: Project Management—Phase 4).

The CNO at this organization has the skills and expertise that she has developed over the years in order to get promoted, so she will initially take on a partial role for managing the finances and all other budgets while Becky learns how to do this. Becky has some knowledge that she had to develop as a nurse manager but not at the level now required in the NE position. The CNO recommends that since Becky already has her MSN, she should complete the Nursing Informatics Certificate courses at the online university where she will have the opportunity to gain further project management skills in managing finances and budgets (Chapter 4, Planning: Project Management—Phase 2). The CNO also noted that Becky will need to understand and develop workflows, develop box diagrams, and monitor and control for quality improvement (Chapter 4, Planning: Project Management—Phase 2, to Chapter 6, Monitoring and Controlling: Project Management—Phase 4). Becky agrees and arranges to take the courses as they work to establish a timeline for her to complete these goals.

Nurse Manager

Ruth S., a newly graduated MSN, is the nurse manager who reports to Becky and as a new nurse manager is required to learn how to plan and schedule staff to adequately cover a dynamic and frequently changing work environment. She has also been asked to manage the budget for the unit, something she will need to learn, as she has not done that before. Ruth has had an introduction to the basic skills in her master's program but not to the extent she will need to perform her role functions well.

There are other competencies she will need to learn as a manager and, just as her predecessor, will take the same two PM courses at the university where she will develop skills such as developing communication plans, learning how to communicate with organizational leadership through report writing, and attending meetings where she will learn more about the group process (Chapter 4, Planning: Project Management—Phase 2). She will learn to develop change management plans and by doing so will learn how to utilize the change process to become more knowledgeable in team building and managing conflict, as well as provide resolutions and manage resources; she became more computer literate as well (Chapter 3, Design/ Initiation: Project Management—Phase 1, and Chapter 4, Planning: Project Management—Phase 2).

Ruth is not well versed in finance so Becky, who promoted her, initially will take on this task until Ruth becomes more conformable with the process (Chapter 4, Planning: Project Management—Phase 2). With oversight from Becky, Ruth will need to review and validate how to assign tasks, as well as delegate, deal with conflict, and assess and prioritize timelines (Chapter 4, Planning: Project Management—Phase 2). Becky also suggested that Ruth work with other peers who have expertise in data collection and analysis, understand how to collect data, analyze and prepare reports for the CNO and NE, define the metrics that leadership will require, and review outcomes (Chapter 3, Design/Initiation: Project Management—Phase 1, and Chapter 4, Planning: Project Management—Phase 2). Ruth will learn how to do other tasks as she takes the courses in project management. Other tasks include the ability to:

- Develop objectives for both short- and long-term goals (Chapter 4, Planning: Project Management—Phase 2)

- Develop and plan "a" and "b" options (Chapter 4, Planning: Project Management—Phase 2)

- Take action and know when to delegate (Chapter 5, Implementation/Execution—Phase 3)

- Define what processes need to be in place (Chapter 3, Design/Initiation: Project Management—Phase 1, and Chapter 4, Planning: Project Management—Phase 2)

- Determine how to monitor and control (Chapter 6, Monitoring and Controlling: Project Management—Phase 4)

- Define the different types of project closing (Chapter 7, Closing the Project—Phase 5)

- Develop, utilize all tools developed, and successfully close a project (Chapter 7, Closing the Project—Phase 5)

Ruth has also been told that the ABC Medical Center will be implementing a new system to document and track nursing standards. She will need to work with IT to implement the system and ensure the system has implementation of standards in place, including a method for documenting employees exceeding or failing to meet standards (Chapter 4, Planning: Project Management—Phase 2, and Chapter 5, Implementation/Execution—Phase 3).

Ruth realizes that she will be very busy at least for her first 6 months in the new job and works with Becky to establish a timeline for all of the new tasks including her schoolwork (Chapter 4, Planning: Project Management—Phase 2).

Case Study: NP

Jill O. is a master's level student who has completed her core courses in an NP graduate program and now needs to develop a project for the two practicums she will need to complete before she can graduate. Jill has found a mentor at the St. Louis Medical Center who will help guide her through her first practicum. Her mentor is an MSN with project management experience and has been managing the department that Jill will be working in to complete her practicum. During the 1st week in the department, Jill's mentor asked her to review some data she has regarding patients with higher than average wait times to be seen by medical personnel in a specific department and to look for specific issues such as lack of resources including personnel, computers, or other issues that might be contributing to the wait times. Based on her own practice and the courses she has just completed, Jill knows what needs to be done when completing the history and physical assessments.

Jill and her mentor put together a preliminary project plan for her practice that the two of them will present to her practicum instructor. In the practicum, the course guidelines require that she first develop a scope document and project charter that outline measureable objectives and deliverables for her project (Chapter 3, Design/Initiation: Project Management—Phase 1). After the meeting with the instructor and mentor, it was determined that she will need to revise her objectives to be more specific and include who will be responsible for each task with due dates and update her work plan (Chapter 4, Planning: Project Management—Phase 2). Jill will oversee the data collection and analysis and determine how the reports should be presented to the key stakeholders (Chapter 6, Monitoring and Controlling: Project Management—Phase 4, and Chapter 7, Closing the Project—Phase 5).

In the work plan, Jill will develop the process for who, what, where, and when the status meetings will be held and how action items will be resolved (Chapter 5, Implementation/Execution—Phase 3). Jill will need to develop a risk mitigation plan outlining the risks to specific patient populations that are put on a wait list and to develop a plan for how certain patient groups will be prioritized (Chapter 4, Planning: Project Management—Phase 2). She will also need to develop recommendations to resolve any issues regarding the lack of resources, who would be scheduling patients, and a plan to add more training (Chapter 4, Planning: Project Management—Phase 2). At this point, Jill does not have the authority to control and manage the budget; therefore, her mentor will complete the actual task but teach Jill how she might do this in the future (Chapter 4, Planning: Project Management—Phase 2). Jill will conduct the resource assessment and prepare a report with recommendations for more personnel and computers as well as training (Chapter 5, Implementation/Execution—Phase 3), which she will present to her mentor and key stakeholders.

Case Study: Clinical Nurse Specialist

Cindy J. has just graduated from the master's program with her CNS and is now preparing to set up her diabetes clinic in the Des Moines Medical Center. She will be working with a peer, Kathy, who has 7 years' experience in independent practice in the clinic but now has asked Cindy to join her practice. Cindy is hesitant, telling Kathy she knows nothing about setting up and running a clinic and she has managed a group only of her own patients.

Kathy tells her not to worry, that she has management experience as a PM, which she gained while in another practice with someone who had a lot of project management experience, and that she will help her using project management tools she also used in the past. Cindy also keeps the course text she used in her practicum that has examples of project management tools to use with examples of how to use each of them.

Kathy tells Cindy that first she will need to put together a plan for how she wants the clinic to run and suggests that she use a Gantt chart (Chapter 4, Planning: Project Management—Phase 2), which will define the days, who will be on what days for all of the clinic employees, and all of the different tasks that will be needed in the clinic. Later, after she has completed the chart and assigned different tasks, she will formalize content from the chart into a weekly schedule, which will be used permanently after the clinic is set up. Next she will need to develop a scope document (Chapter 3, Design/Initiation: Project Management—Phase 1), which will define exactly what they will do and not do in the clinic, and a charter (Chapter 3, Design/Initiation: Project Management—Phase 1) for the clinic, which will define the mission, levels of authority, and other key stakeholders. She will also need to develop a risk management plan (Chapter 4, Planning: Project Management—Phase 2), which will outline how risks will be managed and strategies for mitigating risks, and a responsibility matrix (Chapter 4, Planning: Project Management—Phase 2), which will outline owners of the different responsibilities in the clinic. Kathy tells Cindy that she will manage the budget for now until Cindy gets up to speed and then show her how to set up and manage the budget (Chapter 4, Planning: Project Management—Phase 2). Kathy has already set up a communication plan but asks Cindy to review and revise it now that the clinic is growing (Chapter 5, Implementation/Execution—Phase 3). Cindy will need to set up status meetings after first determining how often they will be needed and the format that should be used (Chapter 5, Implementation/Execution—Phase 3), also to determine how they will monitor and control all that is happening in the new clinic (Chapter 6, Monitoring and Controlling: Project Management—Phase 4). She will also need to start thinking about the project closing process (Chapter 7, Closing the Project—Phase 5).

Case Study: INS

June S. has just assumed the INS role. She recently moved into the role from that of an RN where she worked in the emergency department and completed her MSN with a specialty in nursing informatics. Her role is to help nurses and other healthcare providers by facilitating the entry of patient data into the new electronic medical record (EMR) once it is implemented. June's training to support the EMR implementation will start with a review and analysis of the workflow process for clinical documentation that the nurses will be using on the medical–surgery floors of the MC Medical Center. She understands that she will need to interview the nurses to conduct a needs assessment of the current state—"what are" workflows—then help them to understand the future state or "what will be" workflows, just as she did for her graduate practicum (Chapter 3, Design/Initiation: Project Management—Phase 1, and Chapter 4, Planning: Project Management—Phase 2).

After she has completed the needs assessment, June will develop goals and objectives for the clinical documentation application implementation of the EMR. She will work with Susan, the CNIO, to provide the information Susan will need as she develops the scope and charter documents necessary for final approval of the EMR implementation (Chapter 3, Design/Initiation: Project Management—Phase 1). June will also be responsible for developing the work breakdown structure (WBS) for the different tasks and team members after the team has been interviewed and hired for this project (Chapter 3, Design/Initiation: Project Management—Phase 1). Once the WBS has been developed and approved, June will need to develop a responsibility matrix (RACI [responsible, accountable, consulted, informed]) tracking document and establish the team meeting structure (Chapter 3, Design/Initiation: Project Management—Phase 1).

June understands she will have to pick a number of INS roles as the medical center starts to design, plan, and implement the new EHR that everyone is talking about. Susan, the CNIO, has suggested several roles and responsibilities that she would like June to assume as soon as the final project charter and scope are agreed on by leadership.

Case Study: Chief Nurse Informatics Officer

Susan P. is the CNIO for MC Medical Center, which is in the process of designing and implementing the new EMR system they will be implementing institution wide and at some of the outlying clinics within the next year. She has experience in developing financial plans and the budget to support the EMR but is also working with the chief finance officer (CFO) to make sure that she has developed a budget to cover all beyond the clinical application implementations (Chapter 4, Planning: Project Management—Phase 2).

Her role as the leader requires that she provide support for the PM who has been selected, provide oversight for the project scope and objectives, and identify resources for each proposed application, system, or enhancement (Chapter 4, Planning: Project Management—Phase 2). Susan will ensure that the principles and concepts of project management are used for the implementation of information systems (Chapter 5, Implementation/Execution—Phase 3), which will provide a framework that demonstrates a stepwise process and collaborates on oversight with other leaders to ensure that testing plans are developed, implemented, and evaluated at every phase of system implementations (HIMSS, 2013, p. 2; see Chapter 4, Planning: Project Management—Phase 2, to Chapter 7, Closing the Project—Phase 5). Many of the processes and roles will be delegated to others such as the nursing mangers, INSs, and those who have the required skill sets for a specific job function.

Susan will work collaboratively with the interdisciplinary leaders to establish short- and long-term goals and the specific implementation plans for clinical information systems (CISs) that have been purchased for the

MC Medical Center. She will work to incorporate her goals into the organizations' goals that include the following:

- Improve the clinical quality, safety, and operational integrity of CISs
- Integrate quality improvement and regulatory standards into the CISs to maximize the capability of the clinical data warehouse for quality, research, and evidence-based practice activities
- Work to develop, implement, and evaluate systems and data, and processes that complement the overall system for performance improvement
- Work to evaluate factors related to safety, outcomes, effectiveness, cost, and social impact when supporting the development and implementation of practice innovations
- Work with the CFO on the budget to develop methods to secure appropriate fiscal and human resources to accomplish the work/goals
- Ensure that effective systems exist and are maintained where data collection and information systems are utilized to improve patient care
- Ensure there is an effective project closing plan in place

Susan has many of the skills and knowledge required of a CNIO listed here but she did not feel comfortable completing a budget by herself that also included the implementation of a major EHR for the organization as well as several outlying clinics. The CFO is working with her to finalize the needed budgets and will continue to provide oversight for all of the budgets.

Case Study: CNO

Camille R. has just been appointed as the new CNO with the Medical Center expansion and reorganization. The Medical Center is expanding nursing roles and encouraging more nurses to become involved in administration and leadership where the roles and responsibilities of nurses are expanding and taking on executive positions, which are a crucial part of reorganization. With this expansion and promotion, Camille has been asked to attend an executive development program that will provide her with the knowledge and competencies that these executive positions require to become a successful NE. As the CNO, she realizes she will play a critical role in hospital reorganization that requires a diverse set of executive leadership and professional competencies.

In her new role, she reviews her job description and in a meeting with the Medical Center CEO goes over each of the functions she is expected to assume as the CNO. She discusses how her role is to develop, maintain, and evaluate an environment of excellence that supports the professional nurse and other nursing care providers. She further discusses how she will be responsible and accountable for the overall management of nursing practice, nursing education and professional development, nursing research, especially the implementation of evidence-based practice, and nursing administration of nursing services.

The CEO asks her to be more specific and list how she will accomplish the high-level responsibilities. Camille discusses how her role in organizational leadership requires that she continue to maintain current knowledge in administrative practice and acquire ongoing leadership development throughout the organization in areas where she has had little experience. She asks the CEO to make specific suggestions on how she might accomplish this, given the Medical Center's reorganization. The CEO also emphasizes that she provide critically important leadership by creating, coordinating, and reinforcing mission, vision, values, and expectations that will set new directions in healthcare, especially since the Medical Center is reorganizing.

The CEO further suggests that she will need more education regarding the budget and will need to take some courses since she will have to:

- Participate in planning and monitoring the budget for specific areas (Chapter 4, Planning: Project Management—Phase 2)

- Participate in the annual resource allocations and other project management and leadership functions (Chapter 3, Design/ Initiation: Project Management—Phase 1, to Chapter 5, Implementation/Execution—Phase 3)

- Collaborate with nursing councils, nursing leaders, interdisciplinary teams, executive officers, and other stakeholders including the nurse directors (Chapter 3, Design/Initiation: Project Management—Phase 1, and Chapter 5, Implementation/ Execution—Phase 3)

- Be responsible for teaching, coaching, mentoring, and challenging all staff to use quality improvement and project management principles by setting expectations and planning, and reviewing quality and operational performance (Chapter 3, Design/Initiation: Project Management—Phase 1, to Chapter 7, Closing the Project—Phase 5)

- Set performance excellence goals and directions in healthcare through organization-wide strategy mapping (Chapter 3, Design/Initiation: Project Management—Phase 1, to Chapter 7, Closing the Project—Phase 5)

- Review overall performance including all stakeholders, interests, and operational performance (see Chapter 4, Planning: Project Management—Phase 2, and Chapter 5, Implementation/Execution—Phase 3)

- Ensure that the nursing services are in alignment with organizational priorities, goals, and objectives (see Chapter 4, Planning: Project Management—Phase 2, to Chapter 7, Closing the Project—Phase 5)

- Foster continuous, positive peer review and ongoing leadership development throughout the organization

Six months later, Camille has completed two terms at the university where she took the project management courses she needed to acquire the skills required for her new role. In her latest one-on-one meeting with her CEO, she states she is feeling much more conformable in the role of CNO.

Case Study: Doctorate of Nursing Practice

Roberta B. has been a practicing nurse with an MSN for over 11 years. She is now in the DNP program, has completed all of her core courses, and is now starting her final practicum. She has completed research on the role of the DNP and found that NEs typically practice in a business environment, which requires a skill set that has traditionally not been included in the advanced nursing curriculum. Roberta found that the DNP essentials are designed to address this gap in education while maintaining the focus on advanced nursing practice as well as executive management competencies. In her research, she found a study that looked at roles of a CNO and how the service provided is better and more advanced when the CNO pursues the DNP degree. The report further noted that practicing CNOs in multiple care settings "perceive the DNP as an appropriate degree for nurse executive roles" (Swanson & Stanton, 2013).

Today it is expected that APRNs have technology knowledge, skills, and ability as well as leadership skills such as financial ability and knowledge. Roberta has identified a mentor for her project and will focus the project on the implementation and application of evidence to resolve the problem or gap in the problem she has identified.

In her first meeting with her mentor and DNP faculty, they begin to discuss the design of her project, establish a timeline, costs, and other boundaries including measureable objectives of what she intends to accomplish with the project (Chapter 3, Design/Initiation: Project Management—Phase 1). They discuss some of the tools she will use to implement and monitor and control the project (Chapter 4, Planning: Project Management—Phase 2, to Chapter 7, Closing the Project—Phase 5) with the final closing and evaluation of the project that will be reported back to leadership (Chapter 7, Closing the Project—Phase 5). Roberta's mentor reviews the nine steps the DNP faculty outlined regarding how she will need to complete the development, implementation, and evaluation of her project.

She will first conduct a problem analysis by critically thinking through the gap analysis of the current state/future state analysis or the "what is/ what could be." In the first two steps, a needs assessment is completed in order to determine what needs to be done. She will start by reviewing data, interview stakeholders who may have identified the problem, even conduct a focus group, conduct an organizational assessment, including the mission statement, and review any and all data from relevant websites. Roberta will need to assess resources she will need on the project including team members with expertise and skills in the areas in which she has limited knowledge, as well as financial and other costs. Will she need to write a grant to obtain other monies? For steps three through six, she will then compile all of this information into formal documents called the "scope" and "charter" (Chapter 3, Design/Initiation: Project Management—Phase 1). As the design of her project begins to take shape, she will need to continually revise and update it as she obtains more information. She will need to add measureable, specific objectives to the scope document that will set boundaries and time limits for what will be included and what will be out of scope for this project. Lewis (2007) developed the acronym SMART to be used when writing an objective, which stands for specific, measureable, attainable, realistic, and timely. Objectives are clear, realistic, specific, and measureable actions that move the project toward achieving goals and completion (Lewis, 2007). Specific questions to ask when writing objectives include asking the "five Ws" and an "H," who, what, where, when, why, and how (see Chapter 3, Design/Initiation: Project Management—Phase 1).

Once her scope and charter have been approved, she will need to develop other documents and will need to monitor and track her project once it has been implemented. These documents include developing:

- Project plan
- Constraints
- RACI
- Network diagram
- Cost–benefit tracking tools
- Budget
- Risk management plan
- Gantt chart
- Timeline
- Communication plan
- Workflow analysis
- WBS
- Change management plan (Chapter 4, Planning: Project Management—Phase 2)

Once all of the steps in the first two phases of project management, design/initiation and planning, have been completed, Roberta is ready to implement her project. Since Roberta is in the DNP program, she will need to submit all of the work and documents described to her institutional review board (IRB) for approval. Although this process is not part of the project management process, it is discussed here as an expectation of the DNP program. Since this process does take time, Roberta will need to include this in her timeline. Once approval from the IRB is obtained, Roberta will need to set up a project Kick-Off meeting that formalizes the project start (Chapter 4, Planning: Project Management—Phase 2).

Roberta has now implemented her project and is constantly tracking the tasks and resources in the project to monitor every step in the implementation to make sure it is on time, within budget, and meeting the specific objectives and timeline. She will need to monitor the scope very closely to make sure there is no scope creep that can cause a project to fail. At this point in the project, she cannot delegate any of the leadership functions to someone else but must be very clear on the direction of the project (Chapter 5, Implementation/Execution—Phase 3, to Chapter 7, Closing the Project—Phase 5).

As Roberta completes the project tasks listed earlier, she begins to formalize the project closure and evaluation dates to include the key stakeholders in a meeting where she will review and summarize the project success and final results. She will also establish the formal sign-off and completion as well as define the transition processes as she transfers knowledge to institutional leadership. Finally, she will conduct a lessons-learned meeting where things that might have gone better are reviewed and documented, and a final formal report is sent to the CEO (Chapter 7, Closing the Project—Phase 5).

Case Study: Coordinator, High-Fidelity Simulation Lab

Karen W. has an MSN with a focus in nursing informatics. She just completed a graduate-level certificate in nursing education and was hired to set up and manage a high-fidelity simulation lab at the local community college that will serve students in all of the healthcare sciences, which includes nursing, respiratory therapy, emergency medical technology, and occupational and physical therapy assistants. The community college also plans to make the lab available to local hospitals for interdisciplinary training programs (Chapter 2, Advanced Practice Nurse Role Descriptions and Application of Project Management Concepts, to Chapter 4, Planning: Project Management—Phase 2). The Simulation Lab Coordinator position requires:

- The ability to identify stakeholders
- The ability to develop and measure program objectives
- The ability to identify necessary resources to keep the lab operational
- The ability to create and manage budgets
- The ability to demonstrate outcomes and provide reports
- Collaboration with program directors, deans, and administrators both within the college and at local healthcare organizations
- Compliance with regulations governing student performance as well as knowledge of accreditation and regulatory requirements that impact healthcare practice and practitioners

Karen had previous experience in her informatics courses to enact the role of PM and she has worked to support a virtual learning environment for undergraduate and graduate-level nursing students. She has worked hard to continue learning on-the-job and through extensive reading on various aspects of simulation. She has not had the opportunity with high-fidelity simulation before. What project management content would be helpful for her review at this time? (Chapter 2, Advanced Practice Nurse Role Descriptions and Application of Project Management Concepts, to Chapter 6, Monitoring and Controlling: Project Management—Phase 4).

The dean of the healthcare sciences program has experience in setting up and managing new programs. She has told Karen to come to her with any questions, and weekly meetings are planned to ensure that Karen's transition to the role is smooth and that all of the healthcare science programs are heard to determine a joint vision, needs, priorities, and desired outcomes.

- What should be included in the charter and scope for the Simulation Center?

The dean has suggested that Karen also work to develop a budget and WBS to manage the project (Chapter 2, Advanced Practice Nurse Role Descriptions and Application of Project Management Concepts, to Chapter 5, Implementation/Execution—Phase 3).

Case Study: Nurse Educator

Marcia B. has been a faculty member with the community college associate degree in nursing program for 5 years. She bid for, and was awarded, the position of simulation coordinator for the ADN program. She will report directly to Karen. She will be responsible for the design and facilitation of simulations on a day-to-day basis (Chapter 2, Advanced Practice Nurse Role Descriptions and Application of Project Management Concepts, and Chapter 3, Design/Initiation: Project Management—Phase 1). She will also work closely with all the faculty coordinators across the curriculum to identify design simulations. Her other responsibilities will include:

- Tracking number of simulations per day
- Tracking the number and level of students engaged in simulations each day and the status of their learning achievements

- Coordinating the selection and subsequent use of an academic EHR with course coordinators

- Exploring opportunities for nursing to work with the respiratory therapist (RT), and assistant occupational therapist (OT), and assistant physical therapist (PT) programs in simulations

The ability to deliver consistent educational experiences that can be replicated from student to student and from session to session is critical to the design of the simulation plan.

What project management tools might prove beneficial for Marcia? (Chapter 2, Advanced Practice Nurse Role Descriptions and Application of Project Management Concepts, to Chapter 7, Closing the Project—Phase 5)

Case Study: Providers, APRN, and DNP

As the youngest partner in a practice of three other providers including a physician and two physician assistants, Harry has been delegated to select, purchase, and implement a new electronic health record system for the practice management system. The senior partner suggested that Harry reach out to the Chief Medical Informatics Officer (CMIO) and CNIO and experienced APRNs to gain some insights into ways to ensure a successful effort. What might Harry want to discuss with other members of the practice before talking with the CMIO, CNIO, and other leadership? (Chapter 2, Advanced Practice Nurse Role Descriptions and Application of Project Management Concepts, to Chapter 7, Closing the Project—Phase 5)

The current system used by the practice will no longer be supported after the end of the next calendar year—how might that information be used to aid the selection and implementation of a new system? What project management tools might best keep the selection process on target? (Chapter 2, Advanced Practice Nurse Role Descriptions and Application of Project Management Concepts, to Chapter 6, Monitoring and Controlling: Project Management—Phase 4; Review of vendor selection criteria and assessments)

CRITICAL THINKING QUESTIONS AND ACTIVITIES

Select one of the advanced practice roles from the 11 discussed previously.

Assume the role described, follow the directions for each activity by reviewing the chapter in project management that aligns with the activity.

Reflect on how you completed each task.

- What went well?
- What would you like to improve?

SUMMARY

This chapter provided examples of how the different APRN, DNPs, and other healthcare professional roles might be utilized, depending on the various organizations. The roles include how project management concepts and tools might be applied in the nurse administrator—NE and nurse manager roles, as well as an NP who is completing her graduate practicum project, a CNS who is setting up her first diabetes clinic, nurse educators, and a DNP provider selecting a new EHRS for the practice. Finally, it includes examples of how the project management concepts and tools will be utilized in a newly promoted CNO or CNIO and the DNP student who is designing and implementing her final graduate project as well as other advanced practice professionals responsible for setting up clinical practices.

REFERENCES

Aarons, G. A., Ehrhart, M. G., Farahnak, L. R., & Hurlburt, M. S. (2015). Leadership and organizational change for implementation (LOCI): A randomized mixed method pilot study of a leadership and organization development intervention for evidence-based practice implementation. *Implementation Science, 10*(1), 40–64. doi:10.1186/s13012-014-0192-y

American Organization of Nurse Executives. (2015). *AONE nurse executive competencies.* Chicago, IL: Author. Retrieved from https://www.aonl.org/sites/default/files/aone/nurse-executive-competencies.pdf

Association of College & Research Libraries. (2015). *Framework for information literacy in higher education of interest.* Retrieved from http://www.ala.org/acrl/sites/ala.org.acrl/files/content/issues/infolit/framework1.pdf

Bovero, M., Giacomo, C., Ansari, M., & Roulin, M.-J. (2018). Role of advanced nurse practitioners in the care pathway for children diagnosed with leukemia. *European Journal of Oncology Nursing, 36*, 68–74. doi:10.1016/j.ejon.2018.08.002

Collins, S., Yen, P.-Y. Phillips, A., & Kennedy, M. K. (2017). Nursing informatics competency assessment for the nurse leader. *Journal of Nursing Administration, 47*(4), 212. doi:10.1097/NNA.0000000000000467

Culbertson, S. S., & Jackson, A. T. (2016). Orienting oneself for leadership: The role of goal orientation in leader developmental readiness. *New Directions for Student Leadership, 2016*(149), 61–71. doi:10.1002/yd.20162

Delgado, C., & Mitchell, M. M. (2016). A survey of current valued academic leadership qualities in nursing. *Nursing Education Perspectives, 37*(1), 10–15. doi:10.5480/14-1496

Eliades, A. B., Jakubik, L. D., Weese, M. M., & Huth, J. J. (2017). Mentoring practice and mentoring benefit 6: Equipping for leadership and leadership readiness—An overview and application to practice using mentoring activities. *Pediatric Nursing, 43*(1), 40–42.

Healthcare Information and Management Systems Society. (2018). *Project Management.* Retrieved from https://www.himss.org/get-involved/sigs/project-management

Holle, M. R. B. O., & Kornusky, J. R. M. (2018). Nursing leadership and the future of nursing. *CINAHL Nursing Guide.* Retrieved from https://chamberlainuniversity.idm .oclc.org/login?url=https://search.ebscohost.com/login.aspx?direct=true&db=nup& AN=T903554&site=eds-live&scope=site

Kennedy, M. A., & Moen, A. (2017). Nurse leadership and informatics competencies: Shaping transformation of professional practice. *Studies in Health Technology and Informatics: Forecasting Informatics Competencies for Nurses in the Future of Connected Health, 232,* 197–206. doi:10.3233/978-1-61499-738-2-197

Kenny, P., Reeve, R., & Hall, J. (2016). Satisfaction with nursing education, job satisfaction, and work intentions of new graduate nurses. *Nurse Education Today, 36,* 230–235. doi:10.1016/j.nedt.2015.10.023

Kleib, M., Simpson, N., & Rhodes, B. (2016). Information and communication technology: Design, delivery, and outcomes from a nursing informatics boot camp. *Online Journal of Issues in Nursing, 21*(2), 1. doi:10.3912/OJIN.Vol21No02Man05

Lewis, J. P. (2007). Fundamentals of project management. *Research Gate.* Retrieved from https://www.researchgate.net/publication/31705088_Fundamentals_of_Project _Management_JP_Lewis

Oakes, M., Frisch, N., Potter, P., & Borycki, E. (2015). Readiness of nurse executives and leaders to advocate for health information systems supporting nursing. *Studies in Health Technology and Informatics, 208,* 296–301. doi:10.3233/978-1-61499-488 -6-296

Pope, K. R. (2016). Harbingers of health care information technology...Christine Gamlen. *Nursing Informatics Today, 31*(1), 20–22.

Reichard, R. J., & Walker, D. O. (2016). In pursuit: Mastering leadership through leader developmental readiness. *New Directions for Student Leadership, 2016*(149), 15–25. doi:10.1002/yd.20158

Swanson, M., & Stanton, M. (2013). Chief nursing officers' perceptions of the Doctorate of Nursing Practice degree. *Nursing Forum, 48*(1), 35–44. doi:10.1111/nuf.12003

Westra, B., & Delaney, C. (2008). Informatics competencies for nursing and health care leaders. National Center for Biotechnology Information. *AMIA Annual Symposium Proceedings,* 804–808. Retrieved from https://knowledge.amia.org/amia -55142-a2008a-1.625176/t-001-1.626020/f-001-1.626021/a-168-1.626058/an-168 -1.626059?qr=1

INDEX

Printed in the United States
by Bookmasters

Printed in the United States
By Bookmasters